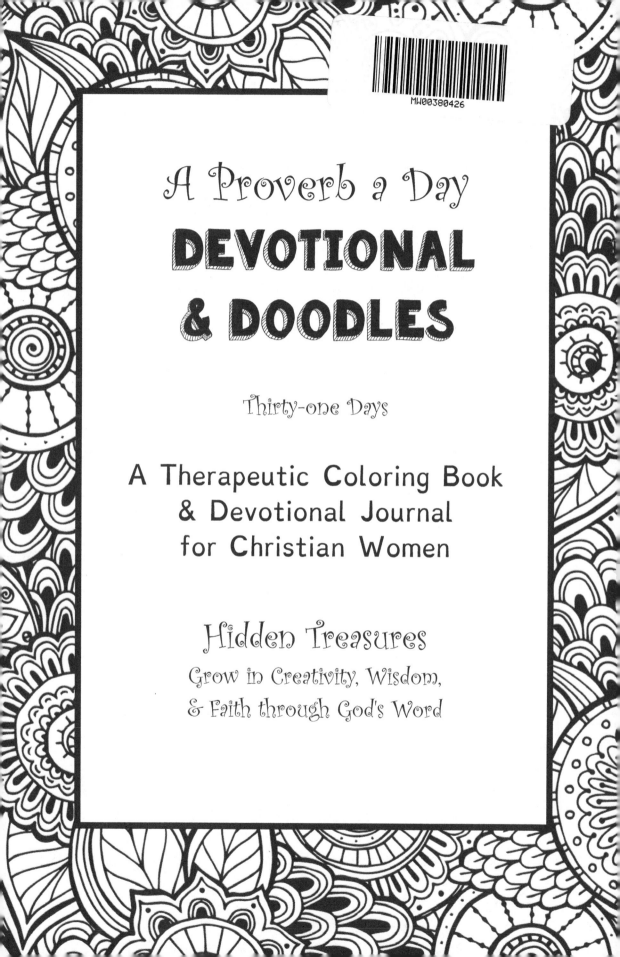

A Proverb a Day
DEVOTIONAL
& DOODLES

Thirty-one Days

A Therapeutic Coloring Book
& Devotional Journal
for Christian Women

Hidden Treasures
Grow in Creativity, Wisdom,
& Faith through God's Word

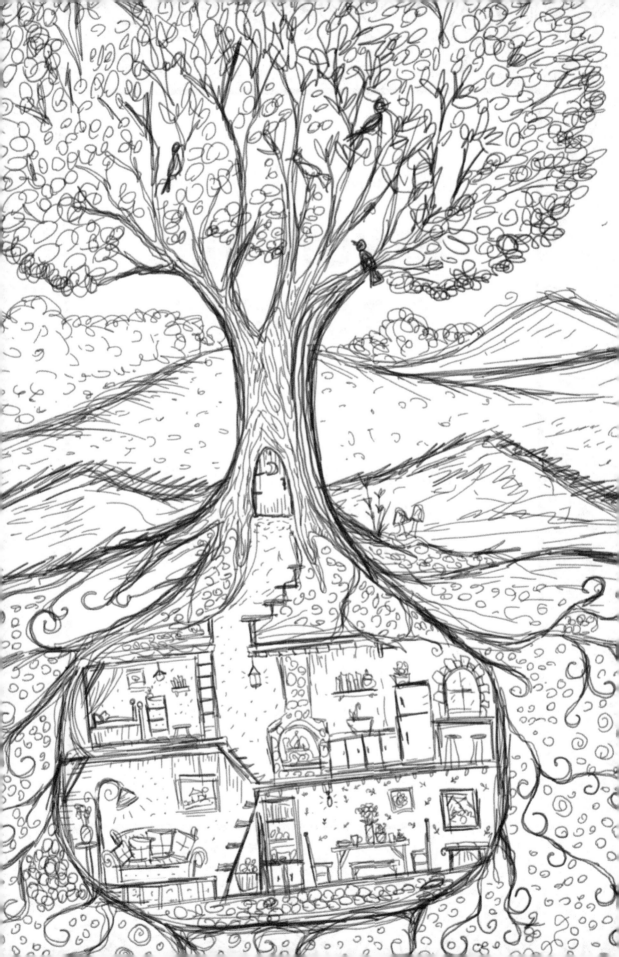

Dedication

This book is dedicated to my children, my heritage, whom I deeply pray will always claim the Lord as their very own. I am so very proud of each and every one of you! And to my wonderful husband, Mark, who insists even though I don't sew, I don't plant vineyards, and I don't get up early without at least two pots of coffee, that I am his description of the "Proverbs 31 Woman". I pray God will give everyone such an encourager in life! I love you all!

~Nora Marie Apple

Devotions Written by Nora Marie Apple
Illustrations/Artwork by Sarah Janisse Brown

Introduction:

A proverb a day. Does it really work? I believe so. Sometimes those short daily "reminders" keep us jolted into the right direction. The Proverbs contain a mountain of common sense. I would not be surprised if the biblical Proverbs are the most quoted of all idioms. They get into your soul. Small quotes are easy to remember...and small candid quotes seasoned with God's infinite wisdom have the power to guide us to better lives.

I once read an interview with Billy Graham who said he reads a Psalm a day to improve his vertical relationship, and a Proverb a day to improve his horizontal relationships. (Vertical meaning with God, horizontal meaning with Man) I've found his words to be true. Though simply *reading* the bible won't fix all our problems, it has to be applied. We have no better source than God's word to give us tools to cope with our everyday problems.

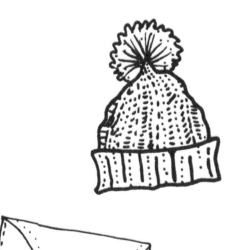

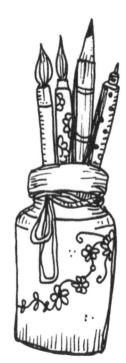

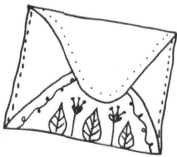

As you begin each devotional, pray for the Lord to show you what he wants His spirit to speak into your life today. I encourage you to begin your daily devotions by reading the chapter in Proverbs that correlates with the day in the devotional. The book is designed for interaction between God's word, your creativity, and journaling. Grab a set of colored pencils or gel pens to work through your devotions. At the end of each devotional, feel free to journal your thoughts on what God is showing you in His word and how His wisdom can be applied to your life.

My prayer is that you draw from His living water, not solely relying on this devotional or any other book written by man. Not only does His word speak truth, it speaks individually to each of us according to our unique situations. Ecclesiastes 3:9 says, *"What has been will be again, what has been done will be done again; there is nothing new under the sun."* This is why God's word is timeless. Sin is sin, forgiveness is forgiveness, and grace is grace, no matter the century, country, or culture. And God's love stretches beyond time.

~ Nora

Day 1 ~ Proverbs 1

Within the Proverbs, we see God's humor. Yes, God is the creator of everything good, including humor. Proverbs 17:22 says, *"A cheerful heart is good medicine, but a crushed spirit dries up the bones."*(NIV) But, as most of us learn the hard way, the best way to live with a cheerful heart is to have the wisdom that will enable us to stay clear of situations, things, and people which bring pain and destruction.

The 1st chapter of James teaches us to have faith that God will give wisdom when we ask. That's the key word: *faith*. Love and faith go hand in hand. In Proverbs 1:7, the word "fear" translates as a word for respect, or reverence, a word for love. As a parent loves their child, they unknowingly impart knowledge to that child by their example. The child imitates what he sees. If we revere God as our heavenly Father, our Daddy, our Papa, we will imitate His perfect love. He will give us knowledge, wisdom, and instruction through guidance and discipline just as we do our own children.

"The fear of the Lord is the beginning of knowledge,
  but fools despise wisdom and instruction." ~Proverbs 1:7

I don't know why, but the second part of this verse struck me humorous. Who, in their right mind, would actually want to be a fool? Who would not want wisdom?

Unfortunately, that describes all of us. Our sinful nature puffs us up with pride. Pride would have us believe that to accept instruction shows weakness. Self-protection and insecurity brings about the proverbial "know-it-all" attitude, which despises instruction and turns us into fools.

Our own self-centeredness causes us to despise wisdom, discipline, and knowledge as stated throughout chapter 1 of Proverbs. In verses 4, 7, 22, and 32 those who reject knowledge are called *simple ones* or *fools*. It's such a simple concept: Listen, do right, and have no consequences in life. Whether good or bad, we live in the consequences of our choices, and also the choices of others. For we live in a fallen world. But how many of us live sinless, mistake-free, lives? None. That's why God gave us redemption and restoration through Jesus!

So how do we apply the instruction in Proverbs 1? How do we attain wisdom? Knowing all about God isn't enough to save; it's in knowing God that saves. We know God by spending time with him through His word and prayer. Romans 16:17-20 teaches to stay away from those who cause divisions, offenses, and your basic drama. Why are we warned to guard ourselves against foolishness and simplicity? Romans 16:18 gives the reason: "*...by smooth words and flattering speech deceive the hearts of the simple.*" We protect ourselves from deception, from things and people that would pull us away from God, and we dig into His word.

Today's chapter also gives us hope. The last verse gives a promise, not a promise that we will be without pain, but that He will be with us through our trials.

"*But whoever listens to me will dwell safely,*
And will be secure, without fear of evil." ~Proverbs 1:33

God is a God of forgiveness, restoration, and love. We are never too far away that God will not draw us back. He longs to lead us, to draw His children, into a life of Joy. He longs for us to experience His love.

CREATIVE JOURNALING

Today's Date: _____

In Proverbs 1, which verse pops out to you? How does that verse apply to your world today? List ways in which you can grow in God's wisdom:

_____
_____
_____
_____
_____
_____
_____
_____
_____
_____
_____
_____
_____
_____
_____
_____
_____
_____
_____
_____
_____
_____
_____
_____
_____
_____
_____
_____
_____

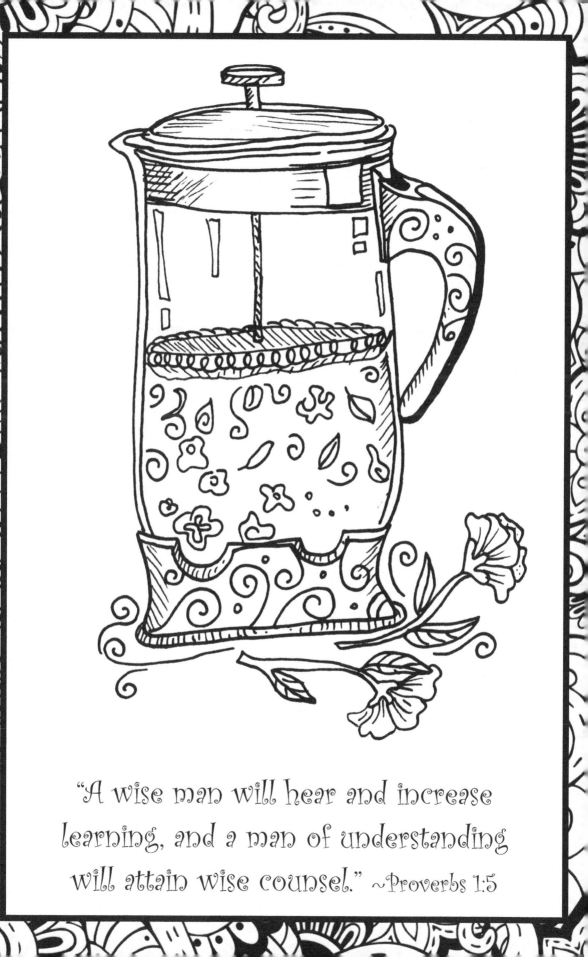

"A wise man will hear and increase learning, and a man of understanding will attain wise counsel." ~Proverbs 1:5

Day 2 ~ Proverbs 2

"He holds victory in store for the upright,
he is a shield to those whose walk is blameless,
for he guards the course of the just
and protects the way of his faithful ones."
~Proverbs **2:7-8** (NIV)

When an athlete runs a race, in order to win, a lot of practice, endurance, and training go into creating the ability to be the best on the field. The game's victory is dependent on the contestants' disciplined life, foregoing "fun" in order to train for the event. While no one is absolutely perfect, the winner will need to make choices that not only will promote themselves, but will also benefit their team. While their friends are enjoying hot fudge sundaes, the athlete in training is sitting across the table munching on carrots. While some things may be good, not all are beneficial. Sometimes we need to say "no" to the good in order to obtain God's best. When we stay faithful to God's good course, we are protected from a life filled with regret from consequences of sin. When we truly believe how much God really does love us, we understand that by saying "no" to the supposed "fun" of the world, we rest in confidence that He has a much better life in store for us. God is always our shield, our guard, and our protector.

"Wise choices will watch over you.
Understanding will keep you safe." ~Proverbs **2:11** (NLT)

We've all made stupid choices, for we have all sinned. If your life is a mess from years of bad choices, just like the athlete that stays the course, endurance will eventually get your life back into shape. Don't give up. Even though a heart change may come overnight, years of habits may take time to undo. Be patient. Live in today. Matthew **6:34** (NIV) says, *"Do not worry about tomorrow, for tomorrow will worry about itself.*

Each day has enough trouble of its own." Start today...one choice at a time. Before each decision, ask yourself if the choice lines up with God's word. If not, pray for the Lord's understanding. Let the Lord renew your mind. Ephesians 4:23-24 says, *"Instead, let the Spirit renew your thoughts and attitudes. Put on your new nature, created to be like God—truly righteous and holy."*(NLT). Even the Apostle Paul said in Philippians 3:12-14, *"... I press on to reach the end of the race..."* Paul had not reached perfection, and he did not look back, but pressed on toward the goal of being like Christ.

"Wisdom will save you from evil people,
from those whose words are twisted." ~Proverbs 2:12 (NLT)

At first glance, the Proverbs seem to be a flowing list of rules, a list of do's and don'ts. But God is a God of relationship. He will never force anyone to follow Him. He gives us all the freedom to make our own choices, whether good or bad. God doesn't want to take away all our fun, he just wants to keep us from the consequences of the wrong kind of fun. Only a perfect God is able to give the understanding (wisdom) that will not lead us to heartache, and give us discernment when deceptive words are whispered by those who would lure us off course.

The main theme throughout the book of Proverbs is seeking the wisdom that can only be gained through the Lord. As you read through the Proverbs this month, take note of the benefits and consequences listed in each chapter concerning wisdom and folly. Though no one is perfect, and even seasoned Christians make mistakes, letting the Lord transform our thoughts with His wisdom by growing closer to God through His word will bring restoration and joy to our lives, affecting generations to come!

CREATIVE JOURNALING

Today's Date: _____

In Proverbs 2, which verse pops out to you? How does that verse apply to your world today? List choices you need to make today. Check which choices are good, better, best:

_____
_____
_____
_____
_____
_____
_____
_____
_____
_____
_____
_____
_____
_____
_____
_____
_____
_____
_____
_____
_____
_____
_____
_____
_____
_____
_____
_____
_____
_____

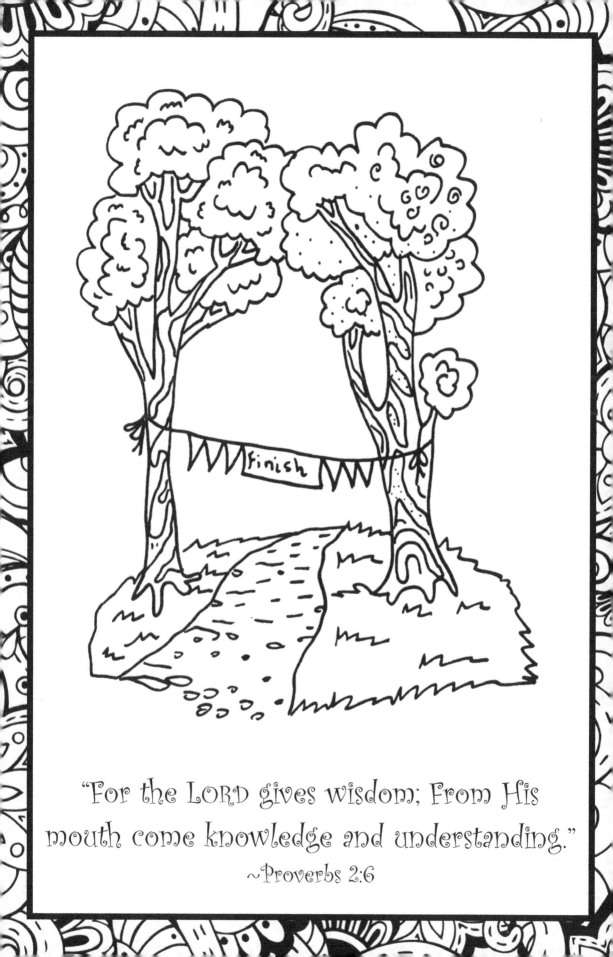

"For the LORD gives wisdom; From His mouth come knowledge and understanding."
~Proverbs 2:6

Day 3 ~ Proverbs 3

Chapter 3 is packed full of great little nuggets! Several verses have been popularly quoted throughout the millennia. But two verses seem to be tossed in the background:

"Do not withhold good from those who deserve it,
when it is in your power to act.
Do not say to your neighbor,
"Come back later; I'll give it tomorrow" –
when you now have it with you." ~Proverbs **3:27-28**

At first glance, the verses are saying to be sure and pay our debts. Don't be stingy. When we are diligent to pay everything we owe, not only do we show our good character, but we show honor to God in our trusting Him to meet our needs. Jesus teaches in Matthew **6:25-35** that worrying is for the birds, *"...Are you not of more valuable than they?"* Figuratively: He loves us so much more than we tend to believe, so why do we hold onto our finances and not trust God to provide?

Yet, these verses also bring up another underlying thought. I like how the New Living Translation puts it:

"Do not withhold good from those who deserve it
when it's in your power to help them.
If you can help your neighbor now, don't say,
'Come back tomorrow, and then I'll help you.'"
~Proverbs **3:27-28** (NLT)

Procrastination is an all too common enemy. A definition of procrastination is to *put off* or to *delay*. Why do we put off that which we are capable of accomplishing today? Sometimes, we procrastinate out of pure laziness. Most often, we put others off out of our desire to control. We believe our schedule, our money, etc. is more important than anyone else.

Both are rooted in self-centeredness and pride. Most of us never thought of procrastination as a sin. We excuse ourselves with our good "intent" of giving, but only when it is convenient for us. One of the first companies I worked for had a saying, "Five minutes now will save five hours of cleanup tomorrow." That concept is not only true in the business world; it is true in our relationships.

Do you have unresolved conflict with anyone? Time is not the healer; God is our healer. Ephesians 4:25-27 says to not let the sun go down on our anger, followed by saying not to give the devil a foothold. Romans 12:18 says, *"If it is possible, as far as it depends on you, live peaceably with all men."* Taking that step toward reconciliation doesn't always mean the other person will respond, but it's our responsibility to do our part.

We need to take an honest look at ourselves. Are we withholding money, forgiveness, or restoration from anyone? Let's give where the giving is due, and trust the Lord to take care of the rest.

"My child, don't reject the Lord's discipline,
    and don't be upset when he corrects you.
For the Lord corrects those he loves,
    just as a father corrects a child in whom he delights."
~Proverbs 3:11-12 (NLT)

The hard stuff of discipline, forgiveness, and restoration only lasts for a moment...the rewards last an eternity.

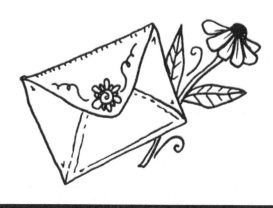

CREATIVE JOURNALING

Today's Date: _____

In Proverbs 3, which verse pops out to you? How does that verse apply to your world today? List things you have been procrastinating and the people you could have helped:

_____
_____
_____
_____
_____
_____
_____
_____
_____
_____
_____
_____
_____
_____
_____
_____
_____
_____
_____
_____
_____
_____
_____
_____
_____
_____
_____
_____
_____

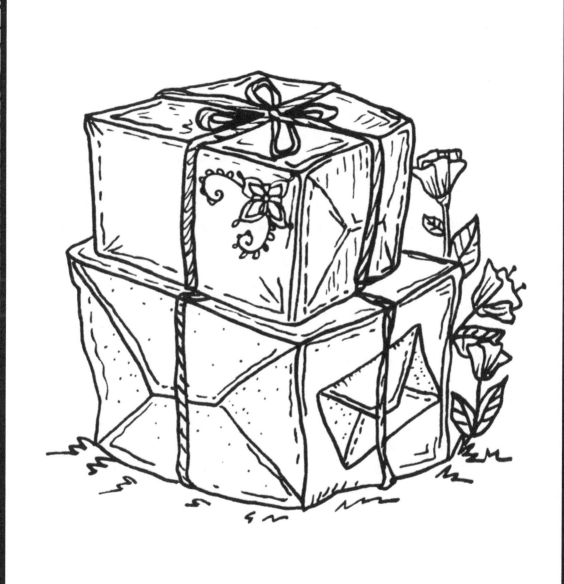

"Trust in the Lord with all your heart,
and lean not on your own understanding."
~Proverbs 3:5

Day 4 ~ Proverbs 4

"Get wisdom! Get understanding!
Do not forget, nor turn away from the words of my mouth."
~Proverbs 4:5

If you read the Proverbs in consecutive order, you will notice a pattern throughout the book. The running theme is to seek the Lord's understanding and wisdom, which leads to God's blessings. The Proverbs also presents plenty of incentive to reject the world's self-absorbed perception, which leads to negative consequences (see verses14-17). It's as if the writer is screaming for us to listen!

"Do not forsake her, and she will preserve you;
Love her, and she will keep you." ~Proverbs 4:6

In the 4th chapter, wisdom is described in the form of a person using the female gender. I love that. Not just because I am female, although it is flattering, but because by using the female gender God is saying that wisdom should be treated as a Lady. A lady should be cherished, protected, and loved. A lady is one who is appealing and sought after. Ladies, our wisdom should be alluring.

"Dear friend, take my advice;
it will add years to your life." ~Proverbs 4:10 (NIV)

Just as a true Lady is prudent, we are also warned to be *very* careful of the advice we receive. The only way to live in God's wisdom is to keep His word in our heart (see verse 21). The very 1st verse speaks of adhering to his *fatherly* advice, *"Hear, my children, the instruction of a father..."* Do we pray for wisdom in receiving Godly advice? Wisdom is based on truth: God's truth. Do we seek truth? The chapter reiterates any advice must be backed in truth or destruction will follow, simply *"Murphy's Law"* and common sense. Haven't we all had relationships turn sour due to someone listening to bad advice or gossip derived from their own self-centeredness? It hurts. Self-serving advice is destructive. Many lives have been altered and relationships destroyed from lack of wisdom by listening to well intentioned advice based on our own desires instead of seeking what God wants for us or another person.

"Keep your heart with all diligence,
for out of it spring the issues of life.
Put away from you a deceitful mouth,
and put perverse lips far from you."
~Proverbs **4:23-24**

In those times where relationships are divided due to bad advice or someone clinging to the world's agenda rather than listening to the Lord, pray for God's wisdom. James **1:5** says if we lack wisdom to simply ask God who gives generously. Wisdom will open our spirit to the truth behind every wrong word or thought. Our job is to protect our hearts from the pit of bitterness, resentment, and hatred. Though we have no control over another, we do have control over our heart and our own spoken words. When others refuse to walk in love, we are still responsible for our own thoughts and actions. Wisdom knows that we don't know all sides. But God does. Was that harsh word spoken rooted in our own selfish desires? Do we listen to others who are speaking (gossiping) from their own agenda?

Our lips have the ability to speak life...and the ability to speak evil. In the end, God will correct all wrongs in His time. We must be diligent to let the Lord handle the wrongs done to us, diligent to keep our words seasoned with kindness and love to others. We must seek Lady Wisdom.

"Wisdom is the principal thing;
Therefore get wisdom.
And in all your getting, get understanding."
~Proverbs **4:7**

CREATIVE JOURNALING

Today's Date: _____

In Proverbs 4, which verse pops out to you? How does that verse apply to your world today? Have you accepted bad advice from a trusted source? Journal your pain in the repercussions of the situation:

_____
_____
_____
_____
_____
_____
_____
_____
_____
_____
_____
_____
_____
_____
_____
_____
_____
_____
_____
_____
_____
_____
_____
_____
_____
_____
_____

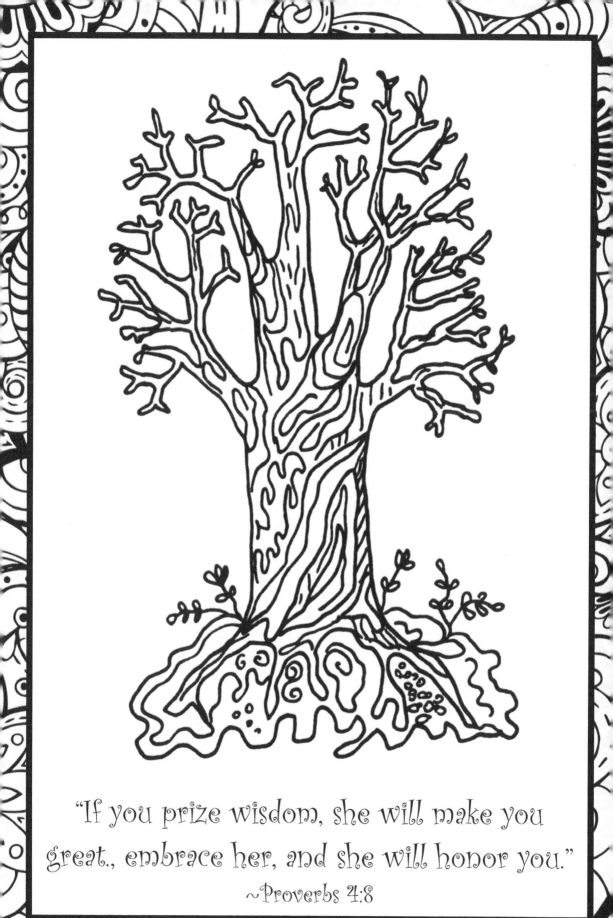

"If you prize wisdom, she will make you great., embrace her, and she will honor you."

~Proverbs 4:8

Day 5 ~ Proverbs 5

*"That you may preserve discretion
    and your lips may keep knowledge."* ~Proverbs **5:2**

The fifth, sixth, and seventh chapters of Proverbs primarily deal with the subject of adultery. Being physically unfaithful to your mate is not the only form of adultery, for God looks upon the heart. How faithful are we in all our relationships? Are we a faithful friend, employee, or neighbor? God is a faithful God, yet we continually fall into our old self absorbed nature. Oh how thankful I am that He is also a God of grace, continually ready to forgive our unfaithfulness!

Adultery is a symptom of a much deeper problem; it's a matter of the heart. Jesus said in Matthew **5:28**, *"But I say to you that whoever looks at a woman to lust for her has already committed adultery with her in his heart."* Adultery begins with an ungrateful heart, long before the physical act. Ungratefulness leads to dissatisfaction, which leads to unfaithfulness. When we fail to keep our hearts satisfied with that which God provides, we fall into a host of sins: envy, covetousness, jealousy, etc. Paul says in Romans **13** the Ten Commandments *"are all summed up in this saying, "You shall love your neighbor as yourself."* Love wants the best for others, and lives in gratitude for that which God has given us.

*"lest strangers feast on your wealth
    and your toil enrich another man's house."*
                              ~Proverbs **5:10** (NIV)

Consequences always follow a wandering heart. When one or both in a relationship begin to lust for something outside of God's shelter, trust is broken and the relationship is fractured. Does the wandering always have to be physical? No. Pornography is an epidemic across the globe, destroying marriages and families, for it creates a dissatisfied heart. That aging mother with all those stretch marks, varicose veins, and sagging breasts can never compete with the airbrushed young perfection on the screen. When divorce follows, so does the division of entire families, friends, and your finances.

"Drink water from your own cistern,
    running water from your own well.
  Should your springs overflow in the streets?
      Your streams of water in the public squares?
Let them be yours alone,
    Never to be shared with strangers.
  May your fountain be blessed,
      And may you rejoice in the wife of your youth,
        a loving doe, a graceful deer.
May her breasts satisfy you always;
    May you ever be captivated by her love."
                              ~Proverbs 5:15-19 (NIV)

Our selfish nature has us believing the grass is always greener on the other side of the fence. Yet, in reality, the grass is only greener on the side that is watered. Do you feel dry and disconnected from those close to you? First, water your soul with God's Word, for His Spirit will bring peace to the deepest holes in your heart. While we have no control over the other person's decision to *water* the relationship, we are responsible for our own heart's faithfulness.

When we seek wisdom in every thought and action, the Holy Spirit is faithful to keep our thoughts pure and our hearts satisfied with His love. No matter what the temptation, be it sexual, chemical, or even shopping, pray for His Spirit to protect your heart. Gratefulness negates selfishness.

"He will die for lack of discipline,
    Led astray by his own great folly."
                              ~Proverbs 5:23 (NIV)

CREATIVE JOURNALING

Today's Date: _____

In Proverbs 5, which verse pops out to you? How does that verse apply to your world today? List ways in which you can be satisfied with the things and people in your life:

_____
_____
_____
_____
_____
_____
_____
_____
_____
_____
_____
_____
_____
_____
_____
_____
_____
_____
_____
_____
_____
_____
_____
_____
_____
_____
_____
_____

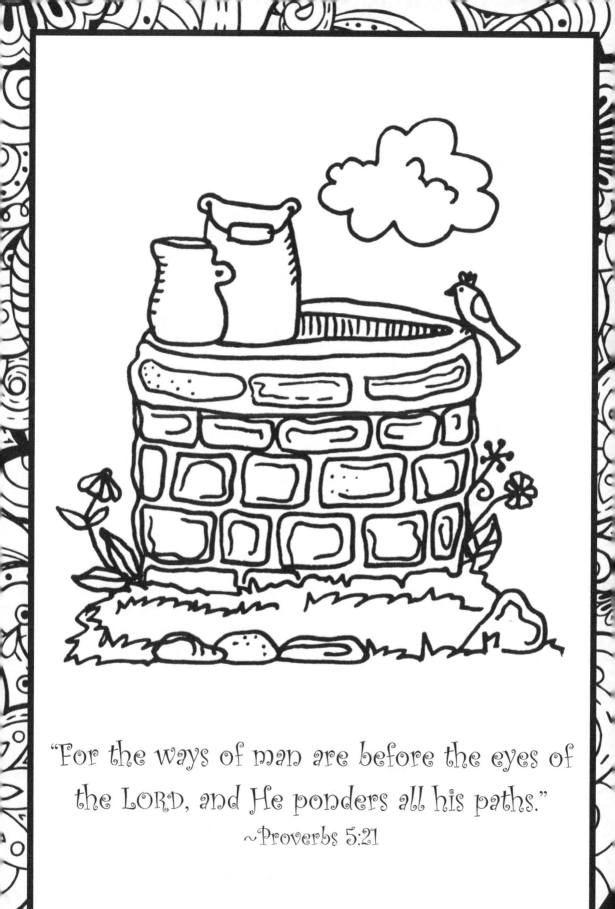

"For the ways of man are before the eyes of the LORD, and He ponders all his paths."
~Proverbs 5:21

Day 6 ~ Proverbs 6

"My son, if you become surety for your friend,
If you have shaken hands in pledge for a stranger..."
                                            ~Proverbs 6:1

A lot of the bible, and a lot of Jesus' teachings contain principles on finances. Most Scriptures deal with the problems we humans have of putting our main focus and our worth into the amount of worldly possessions we accumulate. Paul admonishes Timothy in his first letter, *"For the love of money is a root of all kinds of evil..."* (6:10). Many have interpreted this scripture, along with a few others, to say that money is evil. But, that is not what is conveyed. It's a matter of the heart. It's the *love* of money and the material that causes us to make self-serving choices, not in the possession of money itself. Money is simply something to be used, for the bad or for the good. Jesus said in Matthew 6:21, *"For where your treasure is, there your heart will be also."* Many of the Prophets of old were wealthy and used their possessions for the good, helping people and even nations.

However, the first five verses in Proverbs 6 warn of a different folly: enabling an indulgence. How many parents co-signed on their teenager's first car? How many co-signed on an apartment or house so their kids would move out? And then...how many never followed through with those payments? Many relationships have been fractured due to an unpaid co-signed debt.

We are taught in Scripture that God gives us the responsibility of being good stewards of all that we have been given. In Matthew 25:14-30 and in Luke 19:12-27 Jesus teaches that we are responsible to use the talents that God has given us and to multiply them in various ways. Wisdom will help us to manage our finances to build wealth, not necessarily in riches alone, but through prosperity in all areas of life. Debt accumulation is poor stewardship. Unfortunately, in much of the civilized world, debt is a way of life. We can become imprisoned by our financial decisions, not being able to enjoy the very things we worked so hard to obtain. But wouldn't we want to help people be successful? Are we not to be generous with our abundance? The answer, of course, is yes. However, we also need to use wisdom in how we help others. By becoming a surety, striking a pledge, co-signing, and loose hand-outs we actually encourage the accumulation of debt. Enabling others to accumulate debt encourages the "entitlement" mentality. Most young people today believe they need to leave their parents' nest with the same material possessions that took a couple of decades for their parents to accumulate. How will any of us learn patience and hard work if we are able to obtain possessions too quickly?

"Give a man a fish, and you feed him for a day. Teach a man to fish, and you feed him for a lifetime." ~Old Chinese Proverb

Before putting our own finances at risk by giving hand-outs or co-signing on that loan, we need to ask this simple question: Is putting up security for that person helping to build character or encouraging self-centeredness?

*"Deliver yourself like a gazelle from the hand of the hunter,
        And like a bird from the hand of the fowler."* ~Proverbs 6:5

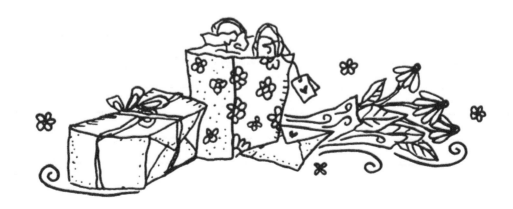

CREATIVE JOURNALING

Today's Date: _____

In Proverbs 6, which verse pops out to you? How does that verse apply to your world today? List ways in which you can become debt free:

_____
_____
_____
_____
_____
_____
_____
_____
_____
_____
_____
_____
_____
_____
_____
_____
_____
_____
_____
_____
_____
_____
_____
_____
_____
_____
_____
_____
_____
_____
_____

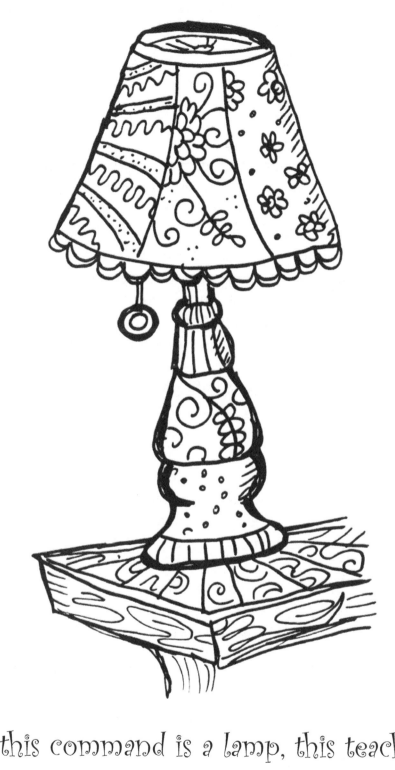

"For this command is a lamp, this teaching is a light, and correction and instruction are the way to life." ~Proverbs 6:23

Day 7 ~ Proverbs 7

"Bind them on your fingers;
write them on the tablet of your heart." ~Proverbs **7:3**

Chapter seven of Proverbs gives a vivid picture of the downfall of a *simple* man. Though the story is about seduction, the principle here can be applied to any area of our lives, from selfish attitudes to out-right open sin.

The first five verses from father to son are a plea to seek wisdom. The terms of endearment used to portray God's commands, such as *treasure* and *apple of your eye*, show His love for our best interest. The plea also comes with a warning to pay attention to *flattering words* that lead us astray.

Beginning in verse 6, a story unfolds with a description of how easily we fall into sin. The New King James Version titles the story *The Crafty Harlot*. While the story is depicted through the male, in my female mind, I correlate it to the old-time carpetbaggers or peddlers selling snake oil. So many of us fall for anything that we believe will take away all our troubles, make our lives easier, and give us pleasure. In our human nature, we ignore the consequences.

"A young man devoid of understanding...
he took the path to her house...
in the black and dark night."
~Proverbs **7:7-9**

How can we blame the harlot or the carpetbagger when we fail to follow our conscience? As long as we live in a fallen world we will face temptation. It's our responsibility to flee. The first suspicion of sin is demonstrated by the *Simpleton* sneaking around in the dark. Is that *thing* we are doing something we do not want exposed? Is there someone from whom we are hiding our actions? *"God is light, and there is no darkness in him at all. So we are lying if we say we have fellowship with God but go on living in spiritual darkness; we are not practicing the truth."* 1ˢᵗ John 1:5b-6. The story of this man walking in the black and dark night is a reflection of all of us when we are out of fellowship with God. The harlot entices the *simpleton* with promises of pleasure, even using words of love. She calls him to a setting that remains hidden and secret. The danger for the *simple man* in this story is with the Harlot's husband, who is nowhere to be found. The coast is clear...

"Immediately he went after her,
*   as an ox goes to the slaughter..."* Proverbs 7:22

He was snared unto his death. How often do we do the same? We fall for something we desperately want to believe is good, and it is available, yet most of the time we don't even recognize that thing as sin. Eventually we reap horrendous consequences.

The last four verses serve as a final warning to pay attention. How do we pay attention? No one mastered the gift of discernment quite like the Prophet Daniel. When Belshazzar saw God's writing on the wall, he said in Daniel 5:14, *"I have heard of you, that the Spirit of God is in you, and that light and understanding and excellent wisdom are found in you."* Where and how did Daniel acquire such a powerful reputation? Back in chapter one, he refused to indulge in worldly pleasures. Though he was mocked and ridiculed, God honored his stand with health and wisdom. Today's hard stand may reap tomorrow's reward.

No one is immune from falling into deception. The same temptations that enticed those in Bible era are the same temptations we face today. The same wisdom that protected those in bible era is the same wisdom that God, through the Holy Spirit, gives His children today.

CREATIVE JOURNALING

Today's Date: _____

In Proverbs 7, which verse pops out to you? How does that verse apply to your world today? How can we keep our hearts protected from the snares of the Simpleton?

_____
_____
_____
_____
_____
_____
_____
_____
_____
_____
_____
_____
_____
_____
_____
_____
_____
_____
_____
_____
_____
_____
_____
_____
_____
_____
_____
_____
_____

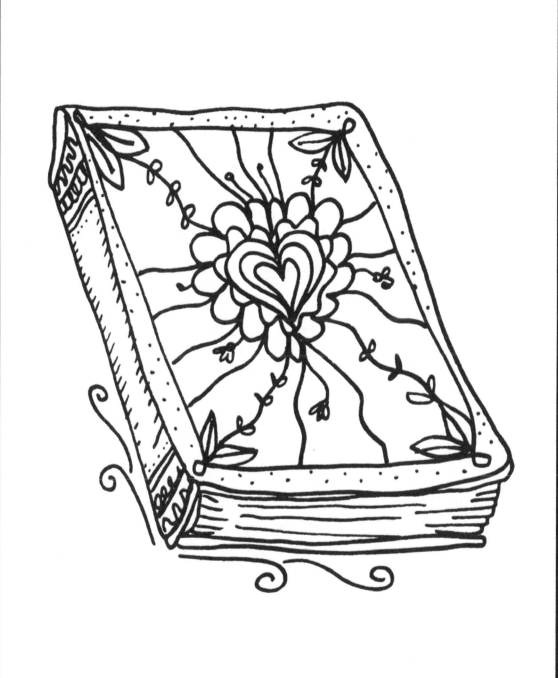

"Now therefore, listen to me, my children; pay attention to the words of my mouth." ~Proverbs 7:24

Day 8 ~ Proverbs 8

As I sit here staring in the page, praying about what God is showing me on the 8th day, I realize this is actually the longest Proverb. The NIV titles this section, *Wisdom's Call*, and the NKJV, *The Excellence of Wisdom*. Of all the subjects written in the Proverbs, *wisdom* is emphasized more than any other.

"Counsel is mine, and sound wisdom;
  I am understanding, I have strength." ~Proverbs **8:14**

Who am I to write this devotional book? I am nothing. I am nobody. I am ordinary. Yet, Paul admonishes us in 2nd Corinthians **1:4**, *"[God] who comforts us in all our tribulation, that we may be able to comfort those who are in any trouble, with the comfort with which we ourselves are comforted by God."* I am someone whom God saved from a deep dark pit. Would I have anything to say that anyone would want to hear? Yet, the Lord has given me more *comfort* than I would ever be able to convey. The woman at the well had received Jesus' *living water* just barely a few minutes before she told about His comfort and salvation to a whole town, and many were saved. But, who would listen to anything *I* say? No, no one would listen to me. But, they listen to God. When God's word is spoken, His wisdom flows out. My weakness becomes His strength. My poor counsel becomes His sound wisdom.

  "I love those who love me,
And those who seek me diligently will find me." ~Proverbs **8:17**

Sometimes the world can be a very empty and lonely place. We tend to look for love in all the wrong places. Most of us grew up with a poor perception of God's love. How could a perfect God love an imperfect me? The concept of *Agape Love* is hard to fathom without seeking God. How can I talk about *Agape Love* without *knowing* God? Proverbs **3:5** says, *"Trust in* the Lord with all your heart, and lean not on <u>your own</u> <u>understanding</u>." The most intelligent man to ever live will never have the knowledge and understanding to know all things. If we talk about theories of life based on human limited knowledge, how can those theories be accurate? But when we seek out and put our trust in the Lord, he gives our hearts peace knowing that an Omniscient God loves us enough to give us *His* wisdom to guide us through life.

"My fruit is better than fine gold;
   what I yield surpasses choice silver." ~Proverbs 8:19 (NIV)

Verses **18**, **19**, & **21** of this chapter talk about wealth. Older translations use the term *fruit* in verse **19**, but newer translations use the term *gifts*. At first glance, our carnal nature jumps at the thought of financial security. We all want to be comfortable. However, put into context, before these verses the Proverb talks about finding God's wisdom and righteousness; after these verses, the Proverb talks about God's omnipresence and blessings. In John 15:1-8, Jesus says he is the vine and, *"for without Me you can do nothing."* One could argue that we can do a lot without God's spirit. Left on our own, however, we follow our own desires which are birthed from our flesh. The *'nothing'* in John **15** is the fruit, the *Fruit of the Spirit*, which is *Love*. Without the Lord, we are cut off of His branch. We are unable to bear fruit; therefore, we have no love. Without love, our spirits are dead.

Are we seeking the wealth of the world, *where moth and rust destroy* (Matthew 6:19-21), or are we seeking God's wisdom, His gifts? For God's wisdom and God's love produce *rich* fruit.

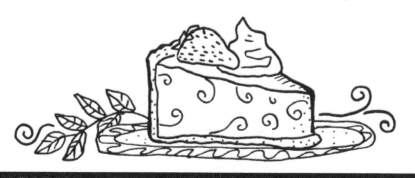

CREATIVE JOURNALING

Today's Date: _____

In Proverbs 8, which verse pops out to you? How does that verse apply to your world today? Do you seek the richness and wealth of God's council?

_____
_____
_____
_____
_____
_____
_____
_____
_____
_____
_____
_____
_____
_____
_____
_____
_____
_____
_____
_____
_____
_____
_____
_____
_____
_____
_____
_____

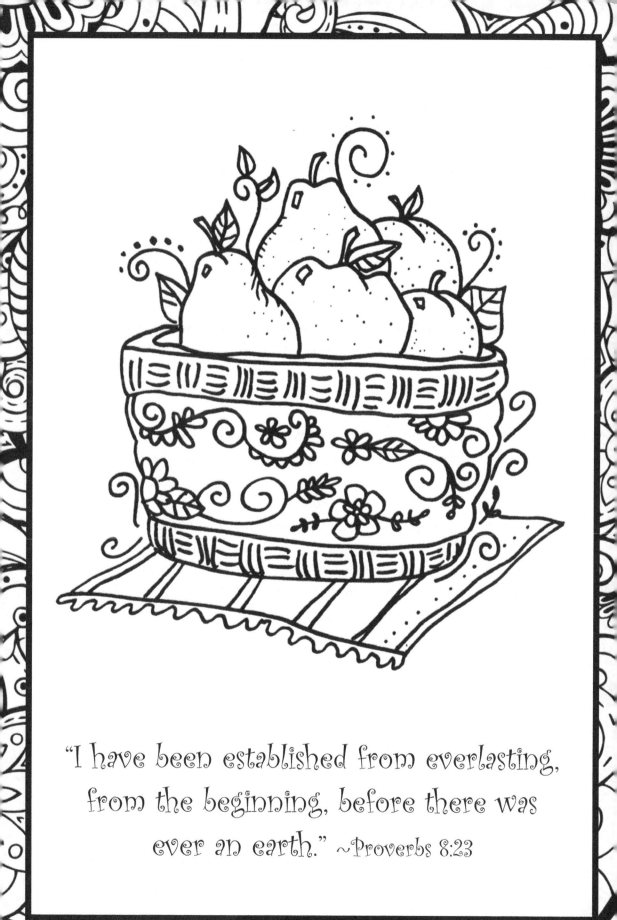

"I have been established from everlasting, from the beginning, before there was ever an earth." ~Proverbs 8:23

Day 9 ~ Proverbs 9

"A foolish woman is clamorous..." ~Proverbs **9:13a**

Clamorous is not a word used in today's everyday language. The **NIV** translates the term as loud: *"The woman Folly is loud..."* The dictionary defines clamorous as: "a vehement expression of desire or dissatisfaction: vigorous in demands or complaints." We are all familiar with this character trait. We have all been there at one point in our lives. Self-centeredness is within the carnal nature of each of us. When someone strives to control others, or entice others into *their* world, they become demanding, and very...loud.

"She is simple, and knows nothing." ~Proverbs **9:13b**

The word *'simple'* as a description of a person is a term that is not used much in our culture today. The term *simple* is generally used as an adjective. We tend to use derogatory names such as 'stupid' or 'dummy'. The dictionary defines 'simple' in its noun form as: *an ignorant, foolish, or gullible person*. The **NIV** translates the term as undisciplined: *"she is undisciplined and without knowledge."* We tend to have compassion for the uneducated. Monies allocated for government educational programs are set up to aid the less fortunate. We make excuses for the loud behavior of the undisciplined as simply being uneducated.

"For she sits at the door of her house,
   On a seat by the highest places of the city." ~Proverbs **9:14**

Yet, in the next verse, she just sits. What do we accomplish by sitting? Nothing. Should our focus be on teaching morality rather than entitlement? Proverbs **10:4** says: *"He who has a slack hand (lazy) becomes poor, but the hand of the diligent makes rich."* Generally, people do that for which they have a desire. If someone *really* wants to become a doctor or lawyer, they will focus their attention on obtaining a college degree.

If a person *really* wants to become a musician, they will focus their attention on practicing the instrument. Proverbs 18:8 says, *"He who is slothful in his work is a brother to him who is a great destroyer."* To do nothing produces nothing. Since we can't live on nothing, we bark out orders, expecting others to do for us that which we should be doing ourselves. That's when she becomes loud and clamorous.

Undisciplined girls are lazy girls. I love to read. I purposely don't indulge myself in a good novel very often. When I begin reading, everything else in my world disappears and nothing gets done. The dishes pile up. The laundry piles up. The kids pile up. I wake up after the last chapter to find my world in utter chaos! Frustration sets in and so does the bad mood. The NIV translation gives a key word: *undisciplined*. During the times in my life when my priorities are in order, and my home is in order, I find more peace with everyone. I have time for those novels when I discipline myself to be sure my priorities are not neglected.

Keeping relationship with God is the best way to keep our priorities in order, maintain discipline, and not feel the need to become clamorous. Are we wise with our time? Do we daily seek after God's wisdom through His word, or do we sit on our doorstep not caring if we grow in the Lord? How often do we follow others who are sitting on their doorstep loudly enticing those who settle for anything easy to satisfy the flesh? Let's pray daily for God's wisdom, and then get up and seek out His understanding.

CREATIVE JOURNALING

Today's Date: _____

In Proverbs 9, which verse pops out to you? How does that verse apply to your world today? Prioritize your to-do list. Is God at the top?

_____
_____
_____
_____
_____
_____
_____
_____
_____
_____
_____
_____
_____
_____
_____
_____
_____
_____
_____
_____
_____
_____
_____
_____
_____
_____
_____
_____
_____
_____

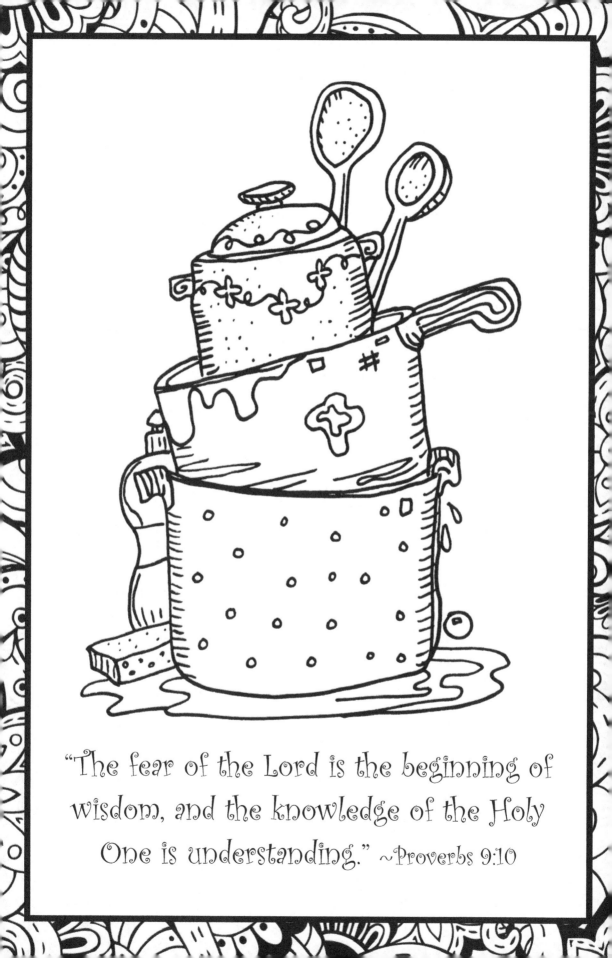

"The fear of the Lord is the beginning of wisdom, and the knowledge of the Holy One is understanding." ~Proverbs 9:10

Day 10 ~ Proverbs 10

*"The memory of the righteous is a blessing,
but the name of the wicked will rot."* ~Proverbs **10:7**

After hearing that a former co-worker just passed away, this verse runs through my mind. Oh yes, I remember my old co-worker. I do hope before she passed that she took the time to make amends with all of whom she was continually infuriated with. My desire is that she found forgiveness, for herself and others. The sad thing is, even if she accepted Jesus and found peace at the end of her life, my memories of her during the years we worked together are that of a very negative and antagonistic person.

I myself have been accused at times of being a grump. We all have bad days now and then. Usually, we get over ourselves and bounce right back to our usual cheerfulness. And then there's that one co-worker, friend, or family member; that perpetual grump who is continually irritated at nearly everything. That one person who ravishes our peaceful atmosphere, thrives on hate, and darkens the whole room.

How will the future hold our memory? Will people remember our laughter, or will they remember our negativity? Will our *Love* be known? The only thing that will matter a hundred years from now is the character we leave behind. Will our memory be a blessing?

*"No weapon formed against you shall prosper,
and every tongue which rises against you
in judgment you shall condemn.
This is the heritage of the servants of the Lord,
and their righteousness is from Me," Says the Lord."*
~Isaiah **54:17**

My Great Aunt Mildred was a cantankerous old soul, quite stern in all her mannerisms. Every family has at least one sinister relative. And yet, there was something rather comforting about my old aunt. As a child, we visited the orphanage she helped run deep in the back hills of Eastern Kentucky. Being young, I believed the stories I heard from another trusted relative who portrayed my Great Aunt as being a terribly unpleasant woman. Yet, when I talked to my Great Aunt, I had a distinct suspicion otherwise.

Years after her death while talking to my Grandma about family history, she gave some interesting insight about the life of my Great Aunt Mildred. We talked about her years of ministry and service to the indigent deep within the Kentucky hills. Not only was she a school teacher, but also a nurse who was responsible for traveling by donkey deep in those hills to deliver 267 babies throughout her lifetime, all without the aid of a doctor. There was no child she turned away. There was no call for help left unanswered. What a wonderful heritage to leave our family!

In God's faithfulness, He made sure the memory of my Great Aunt Mildred became a blessing, despite the hearsay from one relative who only sought to destroy.

Don't fret your reputation. King David often asked, *"How long Lord?"* The Lord's timing is not our timing, but His plan is always perfect...even if that plan or our reputation does not come to fruition until long after we are gone. When we live in the Lord's love, our memory *will* be a blessing. Rest in the Lord's faithfulness today.

*"Hatred stirs up dissension,
but love covers over all wrongs."*
~Proverbs **10:12**

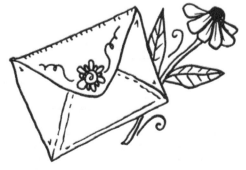

CREATIVE JOURNALING

Today's Date: _____

In Proverbs 10, which verse pops out to you? How does that verse apply to your world today? What kind of heritage do you want to leave behind? What can you do today to begin to make that happen?

_____
_____
_____
_____
_____
_____
_____
_____
_____
_____
_____
_____
_____
_____
_____
_____
_____
_____
_____
_____
_____
_____
_____
_____
_____
_____
_____
_____

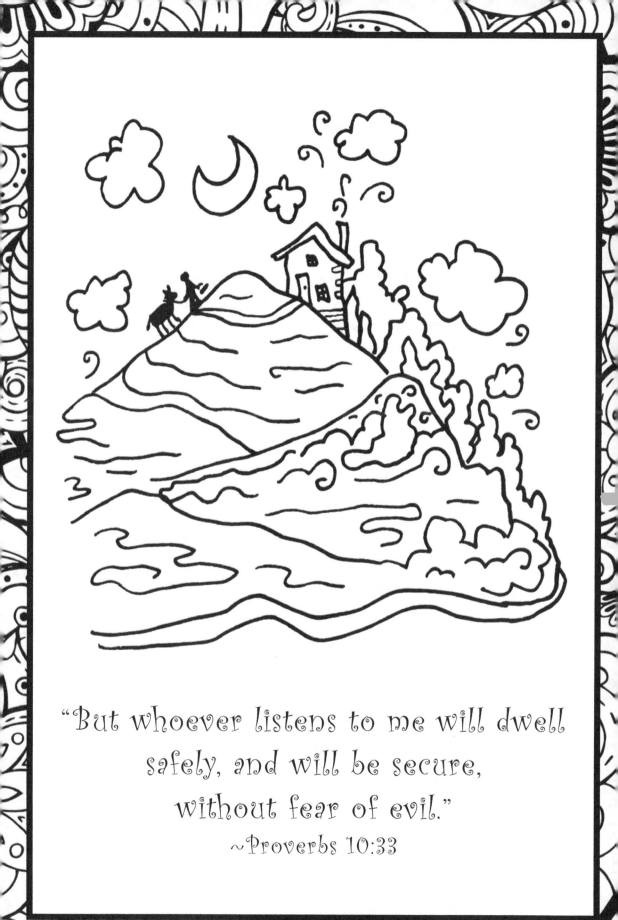

"But whoever listens to me will dwell
safely, and will be secure,
without fear of evil."
~Proverbs 10:33

The 11th chapter of Proverbs contains **31** verses. The Proverb begins talking about righteous living, honesty, and integrity. The chapter flows into finances, explaining how living with integrity will bring financial security and possibilities of wealth. Solomon ends the Proverb with warnings of the dangers in trusting worldly wealth more than God.

About two-thirds through the Proverb, we find a verse that seems to be oddly placed. Why would we find a verse about gold on what the Jews considered an unclean animal, and an indiscreet woman, placed in the middle of verses on finance?

"As a ring of gold in a swine's snout,
So is a lovely woman who lacks discretion." ~Proverbs **11:22**

Most commentaries and sermons I've heard relate this verse to a loose woman, or one who is beautiful and without morals or modesty. Farmers would place iron rings in the snouts of pigs to keep them from damaging the fields or barn floors. Pigs love to wallow in the mire. Before commercialized farming, pigs were allowed to live in the barn stalls of the horse or cow for a time. They were the perfect miniature bulldozer. At the end of the day, the packed earth in the stalls was tilled from the pigs' digging with their snouts under the packed hay, manure, and dirt. The farmer then was able to easily shovel the stalls clean. The pig, however, was always in dire need of a bath! This is the picture given in most commentaries when referring to *"a lovely woman who lacks discretion."* Commentaries describe her as having no morals, having lost her modesty and chastity, the scarlet whore who is steeped in adultery.

Yet...I believe placed in context within the whole chapter, verse **22** talks about so much more. While I believe this verse could describe how a loose and immoral woman would appear, why is that illustration placed in the middle of a teaching on finances?

Some of the antonyms for *discretion* are: carelessness, disregard, ignorance, inattention, indifference, judgment, negligence, omission, and thoughtlessness. These words refer to the mindset of someone who does not process actions and consequences. How many people do we know who fall into the 'dense' category? Sometimes, they are simply ignorant, and sometimes they simply lack common sense. These people are not physically immoral, but make daily irresponsible choices.

One of the most detrimental issues facing most nations today is consumer debt. Recent studies show more than half of all Americans will shop for nonessentials to increase their mood. Fess up girls, how many pairs of shoes do you own? I know women who have thousands of dollars in credit card debt hidden from their husbands. Is there a correlation between the scarlet whore and a shopaholic housewife? Yes, I believe so. Both are based on lies and secrets. Both are adulterous in their commitments by putting their feelings of pleasure over the needs of their family. Many marriages and families have been destroyed due to stress from debt caused by one or both spouses' uncontrollable spending habits. Righteousness is not only allocated to physical purity. Righteousness is attributed to every decision we make. When we use discretion in our everyday decisions, we avoid silly mishaps and blunders that can cause harsh consequences. Pray for God's wisdom to *think* before we act.

"Those who bring trouble on their families inherit the wind. The fool will be a servant to the wise." ~Proverbs **11:29**

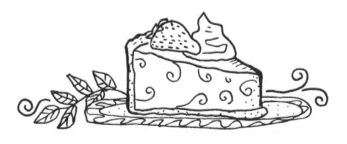

CREATIVE JOURNALING

Today's Date: _____

In Proverbs **11,** which verse pops out to you? How does that verse apply to your world today? List ways in which you can be frugal and honest in your finances:

_____
_____
_____
_____
_____
_____
_____
_____
_____
_____
_____
_____
_____
_____
_____
_____
_____
_____
_____
_____
_____
_____
_____
_____
_____
_____
_____
_____

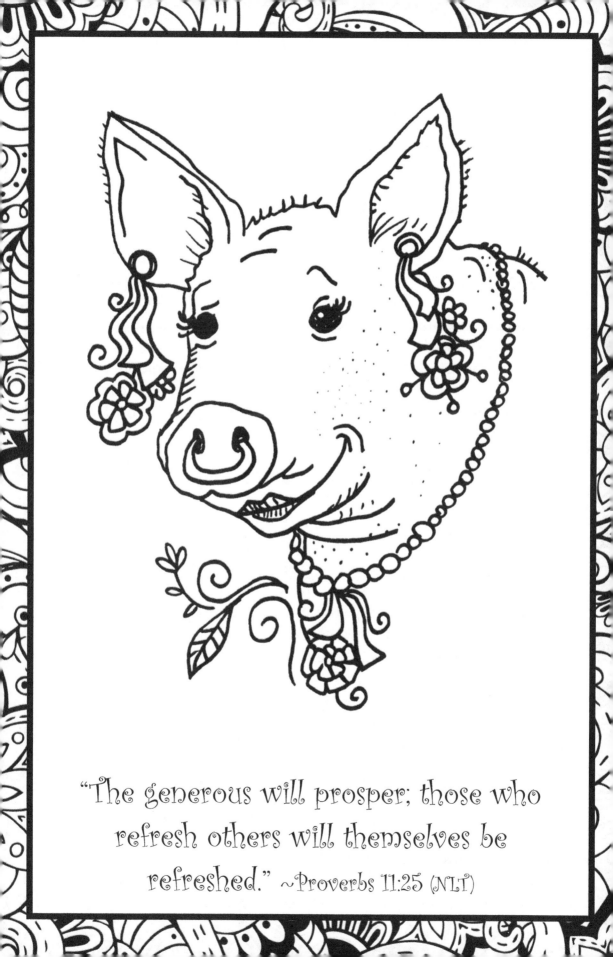

"The generous will prosper; those who refresh others will themselves be refreshed." ~Proverbs 11:25 (NLT)

Day 12 ~ Proverbs 12

*"To learn, you must love discipline;
    it is stupid to hate correction."* ~Proverbs **12:1** (NLT)

The **12**th chapter of Proverbs continues with Solomon's teaching about righteousness; focusing on lying, deceitfulness, and wickedness. Yet, the chapter contains six verses about laziness (verses **9, 11, 12, 14, 24, & 27**). I do not believe Solomon brought up laziness in-between his teaching on wickedness out of sheer coincidence. What is God's purpose for placing laziness alongside wickedness? Our society taught our generation that *anything goes*, that which we do in life does not affect others. Discipline is hard! If a person wanted to live a lazy life that was his/her prerogative. However, the Proverbs tell us that God does not agree with our world view.

*"Crooks are jealous of each other's loot,
while good men long to help each other."* ~Proverbs **12:12** (TLB)

The lie in the world's philosophy leads to living self-centered lives. What happens to that candy bar wrapper we mindlessly toss on the ground or the dirty dishes we leave stacked up in the sink? We cause more work for ourselves, but especially for other people. We develop the "it's not my job" attitude. In the end, laziness leads to the entitlement mentality; someone else will take care of *me*. Laziness is feeding the flesh, which is never satisfied. Laziness looks around and envies that which others have, instead of being satisfied and grateful for the opportunities God has given us. When our hearts are focused on the Lord, we become focused on helping others instead of hindering others.

Being focused on others breeds the desire to better ourselves. Righteousness, however, does not desire to achieve worldly success for our own benefit, but to better access the things that would benefit other people. How many people miss out on

God's blessings due to laziness from someone who neglected to fill a task or a position? We can help so many more people by diligently working toward that college degree, by volunteering in your local school or homeless shelter, or by simply sweeping the sidewalk. How much better would our world be if our rulers, leaders, and teachers were diligently righteous?

"The hand of the diligent will rule,
But the lazy man will be put to forced labor." ~Proverbs **12:24**

God does not expect those He created to be artists to become engineers; or those He created to be mothers to climb the corporate ladder. However, in Matthew **25:14-30**, Jesus said the 'talents' were given to each according to his ability. Solomon said in Ecclesiastes **2:24-26** that God's hand gives satisfaction in our work, whatever work that may be. In Ecclesiastes **3:22** he said, *"So I saw that there is nothing better for a man than to enjoy his work, because that is his lot."* We all labor. We enjoy our work when we diligently develop the talents God created in us. What happens when we waste away our talents (abilities) or choose not to develop that which we have been given? Our labor becomes forced and our life is without joy. Whether we are diligently seeking God's wisdom in developing our talents, or wasting lazily away, our lives *will* have an effect on those around us and on generations to come.

"A lazy man won't even dress the game he gets while hunting,
but the diligent man makes good use of everything he finds."
~Proverbs **12:27** (TLB)

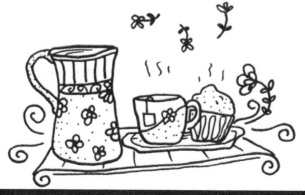

CREATIVE JOURNALING

Today's Date: _____

In Proverbs **12,** which verse pops out to you? How does that verse apply to your world today? How are you working to improve on your God-given talents?

_____
_____
_____
_____
_____
_____
_____
_____
_____
_____
_____
_____
_____
_____
_____
_____
_____
_____
_____
_____
_____
_____
_____
_____
_____
_____
_____
_____
_____
_____

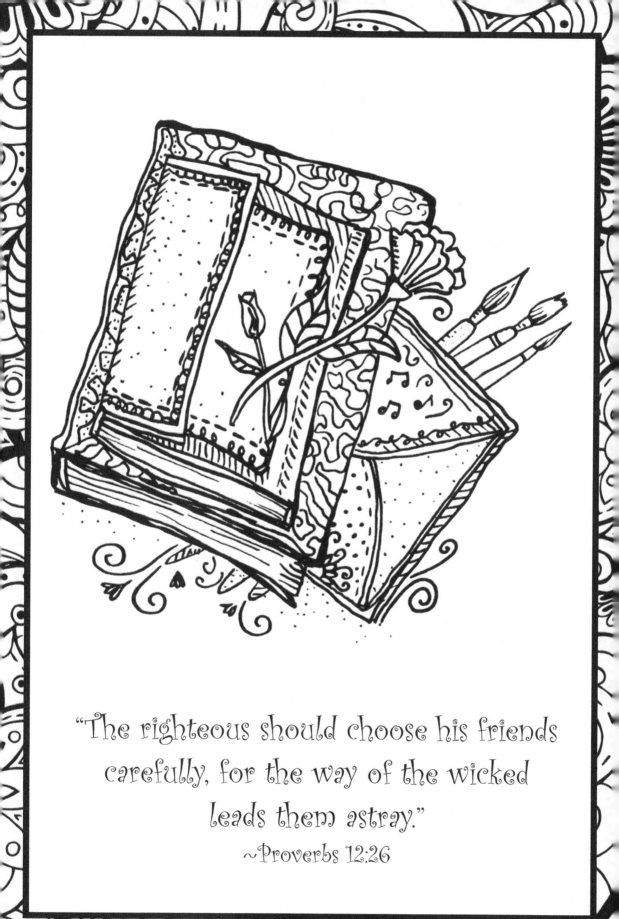

"The righteous should choose his friends carefully, for the way of the wicked leads them astray."

~Proverbs 12:26

Day 13 ~ Proverbs 13

"He who walks with wise men will be wise,
But the companion of fools will be destroyed." ~Proverbs **13:20**

In the story of Job, we hear a lot of babble from Job's three friends; Eliphaz, Bildad, and Zophar. But we don't hear from Elihu, the younger fourth friend, until the **32**nd chapter of Job. In the previous **29** chapters, we see the discourse between Job and his three friends. Elihu finally pointed out that part of Job's attitude problem was with the company he was keeping. Job **34:8**: *"He chooses evil people as companions. He spends his time with wicked men."* Having friends that will comfort us in our darkest hour is a blessing. Though the three friends worshipped the same God, and while they certainly meant well, their advice was flawed with self-righteousness, bringing condemnation onto Job. The three friends influenced Job into justifying his actions. By justifying, he was puffing himself up and diminishing God.

"By pride comes nothing but strife,
But with the well-advised is wisdom." ~Proverbs **13:10**

We need to always be careful not to allow arrogance and pride to cloud our judgment on whom we choose as our close friends. A lot of people believe they will always be the influencer, yet end up being the influenced. We cooks know all about that one rotten egg that will ruin the whole bowl. 1st Corinthians **5:6** says, *"Do you not know that a little leaven leavens the whole lump?"* None of us are strong enough to go through life without support. Life is just too hard. But we need to be wise in those whom we choose to give that support. 1st Corinthians **15:33** (NIV) says, *"Do not be misled: "Bad company corrupts good character."* Ephesians **5** and 1st Corinthians **5** goes so far as to say not to even *talk* about what the ungodly do in secret. This keeps our hearts protected from temptation. Those who don't believe their Christian walk can be affected by the people in their inner circle, consider Amos 3: *"Can two walk together, unless they are agreed?"*

Yesterday's devotional focused on laziness. Proverbs **12:26** says, *"The righteous should choose his friends carefully, for the way of the wicked leads them astray."* How often have we heard of a star sports player lose their full-ride scholarship due to their own laziness resulting from arrogance and fame? Fame draws the kind of friends who wrongly influence for their own benefit. The once sharp athlete ended up wasting vital study time on frivolous parties and activities with no future benefit. Years later they find themselves working minimum wage jobs due to lack of education and an aging body. Sin is only fun for the moment. Whether we are a student or a star, our closest friends help shape and mold our character.

We had a saying back in the day that still holds true no matter what generation we come from: *Birds of a Feather Flock Together.* Choosing our friends wisely can have eternal effects. Jesus always gave us our best examples. He ate with sinners. He socialized with sinners. But his inner circle was twelve hand-picked imperfect people. Of those twelve, three were his best friends. Yes, even Jesus had cliques! The Lord showed us that we are in the world, but not of the world (John **17:16**). Jesus loved all people enough to die for our sins, but his close friendships were not with the unbelievers. Proverbs **27:16** says, *"As iron sharpens iron, so a man sharpens the countenance of his friend."* Are we careful about who sharpens our countenance, attitude, and beliefs?

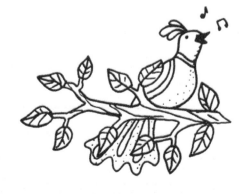

"Evil pursues sinners,
But to the righteous,
good shall be repaid."
~Proverbs **13:21**

CREATIVE JOURNALING

Today's Date: _____

In Proverbs **13**, which verse pops out to you? How does that verse apply to your world today? Are your friends building your relationship with Jesus or tearing it down?

_____
_____
_____
_____
_____
_____
_____
_____
_____
_____
_____
_____
_____
_____
_____
_____
_____
_____
_____
_____
_____
_____
_____
_____
_____
_____
_____
_____

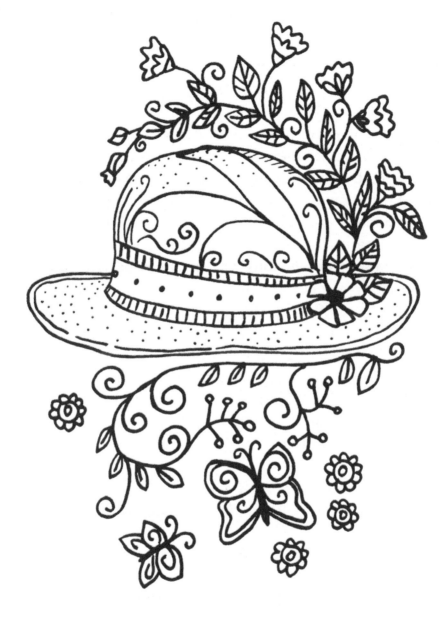

"The light of the righteous rejoices,
but the lamp of the wicked
will be put out."
~Proverbs 13:9

Day 14 ~ Proverbs 14

"The heart knows its own bitterness,
And a stranger does not share its joy." ~Proverbs **14:10**

How can we truly know another person, except by what we see and hear? Sometimes it's easy to assess what is in a person's heart by their countenance. We can assume a person is joyful at that given second by the belly laugh filling the air. We can assume a person is sad, hurt, or bitter when we see buckets of tears flowing down their cheeks. But, can we presume to know the reasons or the source? All too common, seemingly happy people (such as actor Robin Williams) take their own life out of deep depression. We are often too quick to make assumptions about a person or situation before we see all sides of a matter (see Proverbs **18:17** & **25:8**). Yet, in our pride, it's so very easy to assume we know what another person is thinking or feeling. Most of the time, our pride prevents us from simply asking, and therefore our reactions to that person will be unfitting.

"A faithful witness does not lie,
But a false witness will utter lies." ~Proverbs **14:5**

What happens when we assume to know the heart of another and treat them accordingly? If I see someone come through the door with a scowl across their forehead, should I assume they are angry with someone? And then, to top that off, they complain about the blue skies. Should I assume they are bitter or nit-picking? How do we not know that they simply woke up with a migraine headache or have recently suffered great loss? In our humanness, we are all occasionally guilty of these kinds of assumptions. When we fail to seek truth, we are uttering lies. The old Indian Proverb holds true: *"Just walk a mile in his moccasins, before you abuse, criticize and accuse."* (taken from the poem *Judge Softly*, written by Mary T. Lathrap in 1895). Yet, if we walk the same path, even then, do we deeply understand the heart of another?

*"A sound heart is life to the body,
but envy is rottenness to the bones."* ~Proverbs **14:30**

On the flip side, making assumptions on another person's joy is just as harmful. How often do we reject people because we believe their lives to be ideal? We become envious of their happiness while not being concerned with knowing the road they traveled to live in their joy. Often times, we are shocked upon hearing a mild-mannered sweet Christian's testimony to find she has a shockingly checkered past. Jesus says in Luke 7:47, *"Therefore I tell you, her sins, which are many, have been forgiven—for she loved much. But he who has been forgiven little, loves little."* (NIV) Do we rejoice with those who rejoice? Or do we allow our own self-centeredness to prevent us from being genuinely happy for other people's success and joy?

Our heart knows our own bitterness. We deeply feel emotion when we have loved another. People are fallible beings. When we place expectations on another based on our own desires, we will be hurt. People will always at one time or another let us down. But we are not alone in our bitterness, or our joy. Jesus says in Matthew 6:8, "For your Father knows the things you have need of before you ask Him." Why expect strangers, or even those we know, to share in our joys and/or sorrows when we have a God who knows every deep hurt, feeling, and thought we've ever had? A sound heart comes when we let go of our expectations of others and place our hope and trust in God, the one who most knows our heart.

CREATIVE JOURNALING

Today's Date: _____

In Proverbs **14,** which verse pops out to you? How does that verse apply to your world today? What can you do today to bring joy to others?

_____
_____
_____
_____
_____
_____
_____
_____
_____
_____
_____
_____
_____
_____
_____
_____
_____
_____
_____
_____
_____
_____
_____
_____
_____
_____
_____
_____

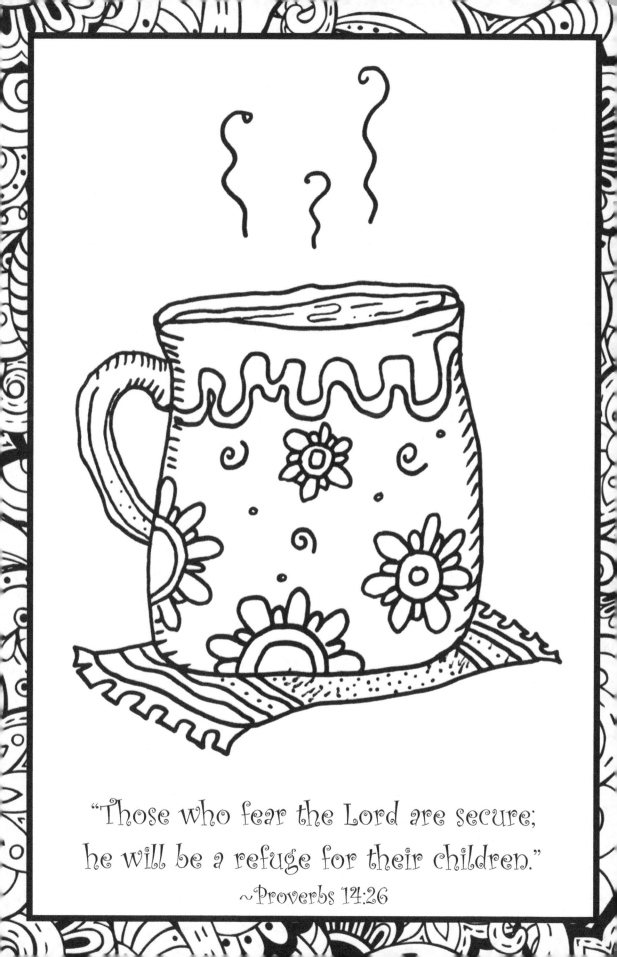

"Those who fear the Lord are secure;
he will be a refuge for their children."
~Proverbs 14:26

Day 15 ~ Proverbs 15

"A soft answer turns away wrath,
But a harsh word stirs up anger." ~Proverbs **15:1**

Almost a third of Proverbs **15** deals with our words. I learned in my childhood the old rhyme "Sticks and stones can break my bones, but words can never hurt me" was far from the truth. Words cut deep. The scars from words heal much slower than any other. The whole book of Proverbs teaches a lot about the effect of our words. Proverbs **16:24** says, *"Pleasant words are like a honeycomb, sweetness to the soul and health to the bones."*

Anger runs rampant in our societies today. Criticism and name calling over nonessential issues can be heard daily from parents, children, siblings, teachers, students, friends, bosses, co-workers, youth leaders, and even pastors. Did I miss anyone? You? Me? Proverbs **26:18-19** in the Message says: *"People who shrug off deliberate deceptions, saying, "I didn't mean it, I was only joking," are worse than careless campers who walk away from smoldering campfires."* Criticism, coarse joking, and put-downs out of your own insecurity are easy habits to develop. A harsh word knows no social boundary. Scoffers can be found in all walks of life, in any ethnic group.

Definition of *Wrath*: strong, stern, or fierce anger; deeply resentful indignation; vengeance or punishment as the consequence of anger.

Jesus chastised the Pharisees in Matthew **12:34** saying, *"Brood of vipers! How can you, being evil, speak good things? For out of the abundance of the heart the mouth speaks."* Jesus was going around doing good works and they felt their position was threatened by his presence. Through their insecurity, they accused the Lord of wrong doing. Their envy, jealousy, and pride, turned into wrath. While presenting a good image on the outside, God knew the wrath in their hearts. He knows all our hearts.

"A wholesome tongue is a tree of life,
but perverseness in it breaks the spirit." ~Proverbs **15:4**

What makes a person spew out wrath? Usually the source of the anger flowing out comes from deep within and has nothing to do with the poor recipient. Galatians **5:22-23** says, *"But the fruit of the Spirit is love, joy, peace, longsuffering, kindness, goodness, faithfulness, gentleness, self-control."* If the heart is at peace, our words will reflect life. If the heart is hard, lost, or full of envy, it will be void of love. When someone projects their anger or wrath towards us, before taking their words personally, we should seek to find the source. They may need understanding, compassion, or grace from Jesus for a broken spirit.

"A wrathful man stirs up strife,
but he who is slow to anger allays contention." ~Proverbs **15:18**

Our own wrath will damage our relationships, not only with people, but with God. Our anger causes us to distance ourselves from anything good. Hurt people hurt people. In those times where you turn down that road of wrath, pray for God to calm your spirit. He will. Practice patience, which dispels wrath. Try to understand others before reacting out of your flesh. Learning how to respond with patience and kindness will dispel wrath and turn around a bad situation.

"Come to Me, all you who labor and are heavy laden, and I will give you rest. Take My yoke upon you and learn from Me, for I am gentle and lowly in heart, and you will find rest for your souls. For My yoke is easy and My burden is light."
~Matthew **11:28-30**

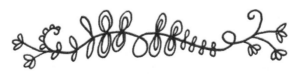

CREATIVE JOURNALING

Today's Date: _____

In Proverbs **15**, which verse pops out to you? How does that verse apply to your world today? List ways in which you can use your words to build each other up:

_____
_____
_____
_____
_____
_____
_____
_____
_____
_____
_____
_____
_____
_____
_____
_____
_____
_____
_____
_____
_____
_____
_____
_____
_____
_____
_____
_____
_____
_____
_____

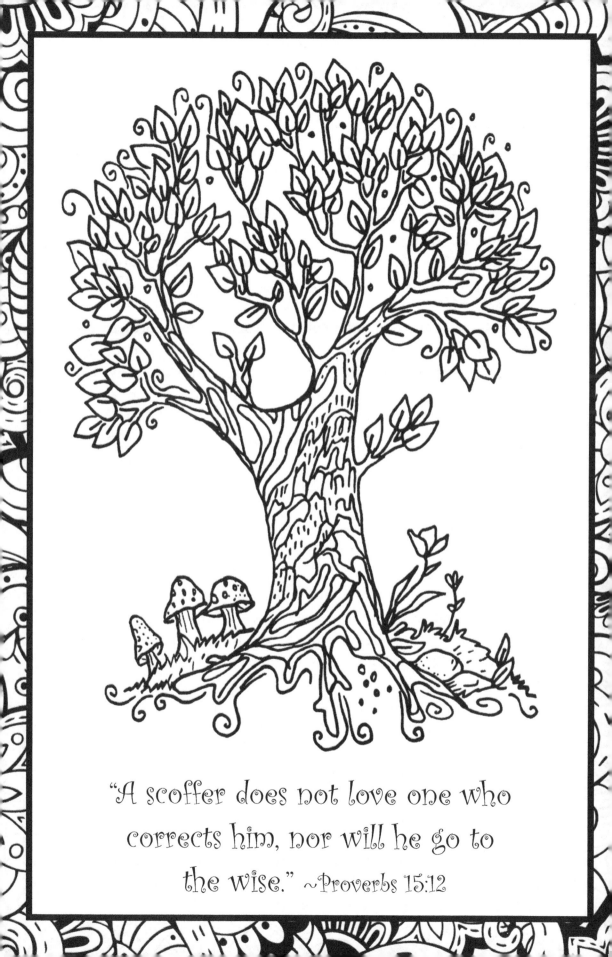

"A scoffer does not love one who corrects him, nor will he go to the wise." ~Proverbs 15:12

Day 16 ~ Proverbs 16

*"The preparations of the heart belong to man,
But the answer of the tongue is from the Lord."* ~Proverbs **16:1**

Pride is such an ugly character. Some say pride is the original sin. It was pride that entered Lucifer's heart and puffed him up so high he was cast out of heaven (see Ezekiel **28:11-19** and Isaiah **14:12-15**). Most commentaries mention Balaam, the soothsayer, in their writings on pride (see Numbers **23**). Here, in Proverbs **16**, we can see that in the first verse. Balaam believed God could be manipulated for his own profit. After Balaam was hired for divination to curse God's people, an Angel was sent to kill Balaam when he did not obey God's warning. After beating his donkey for refusing to go forward, God opened the mouth of the donkey to speak to Balaam. That would surely get my attention! The funny thing is, Balaam talked back to the donkey! We don't realize how ridiculous we look when we are heaped in sin.

*"Pride goes before destruction,
    And a haughty spirit before a fall."* ~Proverbs **16:18**

Unfortunately, like Balaam, most of us try to walk with one foot on the right road and the other foot on the left. We present ourselves as being righteous, following all the rules, wearing the latest fashions, while our hearts are black. In our pride, we believe we are in control. We believe, like Balaam, we can manipulate God. In the end, Balaam did not profit from his actions and ultimately died by the sword.

*"All the ways of a man are pure in his own eyes,
    But the Lord weighs the spirits."* ~Proverbs **16:2**

Sometimes pride is confused with satisfaction. My sheets are folded to such perfection that they could be put back in the original store packaging. The project for the company's new product was so successful that I received a promotion. I take great satisfaction in an accomplishment (see Ecclesiastes 3:9-13). However, that satisfaction morphs into pride when I fall into the belief that my accomplishments are better and higher than others. Our spirits are opened up to self-centered attitudes that demean those around us. We tend to forget that we are but mere specks in the universe. His word teaches us not to compare ourselves with others or to think we are better than anyone else. Galatians 6:2-5 says, *"Bear one another's burdens, and so fulfill the law of Christ. For if anyone thinks himself to be something, when he is nothing, he deceives himself. But let each one examine his own work, and then he will have rejoicing in himself alone, and not in another. For each one shall bear his own load."*

Do we live in humility?

"A man's heart plans his way,
    But the Lord directs his steps."
                    ~Proverbs 16:9

Ultimately, we have two roads in life: the road of humility or the road of pride. Most of us fail to consider the consequences to those roads. Why wouldn't we take the road to righteousness and humility? Pride. Hanging on to the belief that we know-it-all and rejecting a perfect God's guidance assures we will live with the consequences of our mistakes. Without the consequences of sin, we have no baggage and no regrets. The Lord will always bring about our good. Romans 8:28 says, *"And we know that all things work together for good..."* We find peace in allowing God to direct our steps. Even for those who find themselves heaped in regret, God is a God of restoration. It's never too late to let go of your pride and begin to let the Lord direct your steps, letting His love fill your heart, bringing peace to your world.

"The silver-haired head is a crown of glory,
    If it is found in the way of righteousness."
                    ~Proverbs 16:31

CREATIVE JOURNALING

Today's Date: _____

In Proverbs 16, which verse pops out to you? How does that verse apply to your world today? What ways have you allowed pride to influence your thoughts?

_____
_____
_____
_____
_____
_____
_____
_____
_____
_____
_____
_____
_____
_____
_____
_____
_____
_____
_____
_____
_____
_____
_____
_____
_____
_____
_____
_____
_____
_____

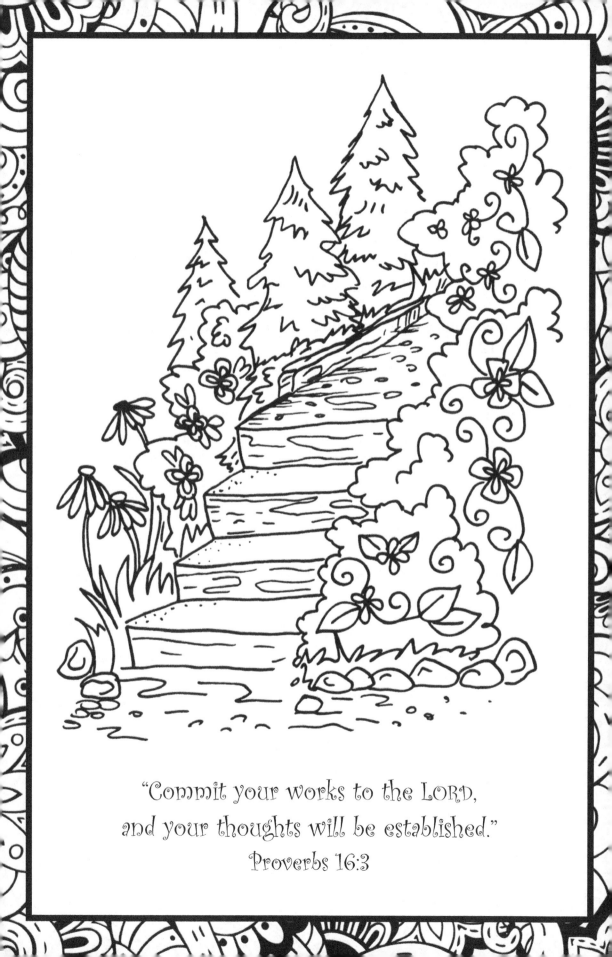

"Commit your works to the LORD,
and your thoughts will be established."
Proverbs 16:3

"Better is a dry morsel with quietness,
Than a house full of feasting with strife."
~Proverbs **17:1**

At least six verses of Proverbs 17 speak directly to the family. King David is my hero! I love reading in 1st and 2nd Samuel the account of David's life. My spirit is lifted and heightened every time I read David's Psalms. More than anyone who ever lived, David was attributed as a man after God's own heart. Yet, because of King David's own sins (2nd Samuel **12:10**), the sword never left his house. His was one of the most dysfunctional families in history. His wives were... well, he had way too many cooks in the same kitchen. His children lied, cheated, stole, raped, and murdered...each other! Absalom, his oldest son, conspired to overthrow the kingdom and kill his own father. If Hollywood were to film the actual events of David's life the movie would be released with an "R" rating or worse! His children grew up in wealth, yet had more drama than a soap-opera!

"A foolish son is a grief to his father,
And bitterness to her who bore him."
~Proverbs **17:25**

Though King David saw his children make horrible decisions, even unto death, he grieved for his children. David recognized in 2nd Samuel **16:5-14** that the calamity he experienced was due to his own sin; calamity prophesied by the Prophet Nathan in chapter **12**. The Apostle Paul admonishes fathers in Ephesians **6:4**, *"And you, fathers, do not provoke your children to wrath, but bring them up in the training and admonition of the Lord."* Children learn as the example they are given, not the words spoken. The Jamieson-Fausset-Brown Bible Commentary states: *"The fathers are specified as being the fountains of domestic authority. Fathers are more prone to* passion in relation to their children than mothers, whose fault is rather over-indulgence." Fathers, do you project anger or ridicule your children? Then you can't be upset if they show outbursts of anger. Mothers, do you belittle or lie to or about your children? Then you can't be upset when they despise you. Do we project indifference to our children? Then we can't be upset if they show indifference to our beliefs. This is what King David experienced. He was busy elsewhere. He showed his children contradiction. As a result, they rebelled, bringing humiliation and destruction to their own family.

"He who begets a scoffer does so to his sorrow,
  And the father of a fool has no joy."
         ~Proverbs 17:21

The dictionary describes scoffer as; someone who expresses mockery, derision, doubt, or derisive scorn; to jeer. We all occasionally fail. Do you fall into that category? Out of your own insecurity, do you make fun of others in hopes to elevate yourself? When your derogatory jabs are questioned, do you laughingly claim the recipient of your mockery is too sensitive and you were only joking? I don't believe people realize their own divisiveness. When a family falls into the habit of squabbling, no meal is joyful. Sometimes, the test of Christian love is greater within our own families. Oh to love with the love of 1st Corinthians 13; *"Love suffers long and is kind; love does not envy; love does not parade itself, is not puffed up; does not behave rudely, does not seek its own, is not provoked, thinks no evil; does not rejoice in iniquity, but rejoices in the truth; bears all things, believes all things, hopes all things, endures all things."*

What would happen in our families if we took just one of these attributes? Kindness? Truth? Hope? Love?

"Children's children are the crown of old men,
    And the glory of children is their father."
                   ~Proverbs 17:6

CREATIVE JOURNALING

Today's Date: _____

In Proverbs 17, which verse pops out to you? How does that verse apply to your world today? Journal about your family dinners as a child, whether good or bad:

_____
_____
_____
_____
_____
_____
_____
_____
_____
_____
_____
_____
_____
_____
_____
_____
_____
_____
_____
_____
_____
_____
_____
_____
_____
_____
_____
_____
_____

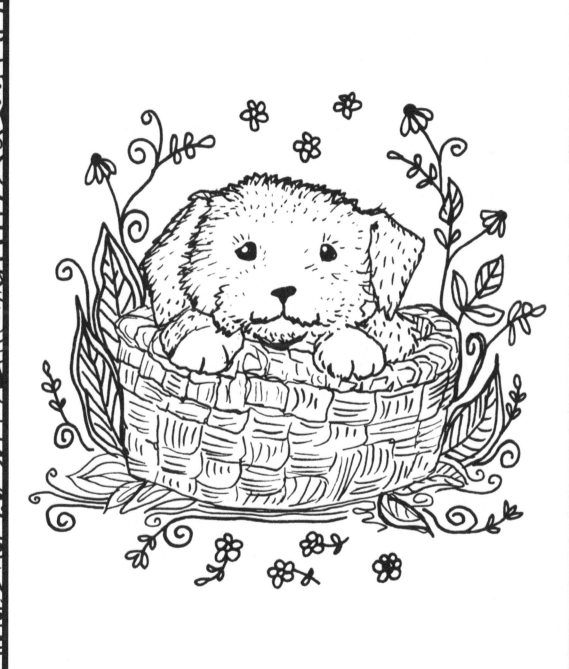

"The refining pot is for silver and the furnace for gold, but the LORD tests the hearts." ~Proverbs 17:3

Day 18 ~ Proverbs 18

Law enforcement officers are trained to take statements from every possible witness before writing up a report. The Officers look at all angles before stating their conclusions. Essentially, they unknowingly follow the principles written centuries ago in our Bible:

*"He who states his case first seems right,
    until his rival comes and cross-examines him."*
                                                    ~Proverbs **18:17** (AMP)

Upon hearing a loud bang, we looked outside our window to see two crashed vehicles on the other side of the road. The teenage boy who side-swiped the oncoming truck by crossing the center-line was a fairly new driver. I felt sorry and glad for him at the same time. While it's never good to be in any accident, sometimes, especially for boys, having a non-injury accident early on teaches hard lessons in humility.

The first-hand account from the second vehicle following the youth claimed he was trying to pass another vehicle. Of this, the witness was certain of what he saw. Yet, after the Officer interviewed *all* witnesses, it was determined there was no vehicle in front of the youth for him to pass. Admittedly, the very embarrassed youth lost control while reaching in the passenger's seat for his hair brush.

Do we look at all sides in our relationships? Do we really know what it is we think we know? Maybe, just maybe, we should at least ask? Would we want others to do the same for us? In our relationships, Jesus taught in Matthew 18:15-17 we are to first go privately to the one who wronged us, and then we are to take two or three to establish a witness. Paul teaches in 2nd Corinthians **13:1**, 1st Timothy **5:19**; and in Hebrews **10:28**, not to bring an accusation against anyone without two or three witnesses. That *second set of eyes* often times will give a different perspective that can bring healing to any relationship.

Comparable to the police at the accident scene, we also need to weigh the evidence and not rely on heresy. We need to pray for wisdom and discernment to be alert to any dishonesty. At the trial of Jesus: *"The chief priests and the whole Sanhedrin were looking for false evidence against Jesus so that they could put him to death. But they did not find any, though many false witnesses came forward."* ~Matthew 26:59-60 (NIV) Did you catch that? Even though a lot of people testified against him, they could not find *evidence* to collaborate their stories.

"Death and life are in the power of the tongue,
And those who love it will eat its fruit." ~Proverbs 18:21

When you hear a *sob* story, are you listening to an opinion or the evidence of actual events? How many relationships have been destroyed by good but gullible people not verifying stories heard from so-called 'trusted' sources? We hear the hurt and perceived pain in their voices as the storytellers recount events that describe injustices done, and we want to defend our loved ones and friends against the so-called *evil* inflicted on them. Why would we question their side of the issues? After all, they are our best friend, our teacher, our pastor, our mentor, our parent. Why would we question? We question because we live in a fallible world. We are all one-sided human beings. We react and feel based on *our* own experiences. And maybe, just maybe, even the storyteller does not know the other side. A wise one is never gullible.

"He who answers a matter before he hears it, it is folly and shame to him."

~Proverbs 18:13

CREATIVE JOURNALING

Today's Date: _____

In Proverbs 18, which verse pops out to you? How does that verse apply to your world today? Do you have any situations that need clarity and God's wisdom?

_____
_____
_____
_____
_____
_____
_____
_____
_____
_____
_____
_____
_____
_____
_____
_____
_____
_____
_____
_____
_____
_____
_____
_____
_____
_____
_____

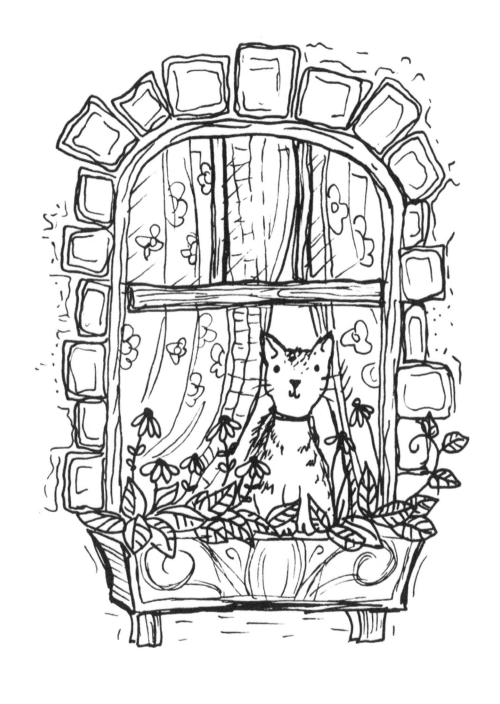

"A fool has no delight in understanding,
but in expressing his own heart."
~Proverbs 18:2

*"Houses and riches are an inheritance from fathers,
but a prudent wife is from the Lord."* ~Proverbs **19:14**

Does our world respect the marriage union? An antonym for prudent is reckless, which is a lack of self-control based in self-centeredness. To be prudent is to be careful, cautious, and wise.

God said in Genesis **2:24** *"the two shall be one."* How can a couple be "one" unit if their Love Tanks are being filled outside the marriage? Love is to want the best for the other person and leave our desires aside. Paul said in Ephesians **5:25** (NLT) *"For husbands, this means love your wives, just as Christ loved the church. He gave up his life for her."* Now, I don't believe he meant for husbands to physically die, but rather to give up his desires, dreams, and wants; to replace his personal (self) desires with a desire for his marriage as a unit. And, yes, that's easier said than done...especially in our world. It's no different for women. Our first priority is to God, then our family...our immediate family. (God also said to leave our parents!)

How can we identify a lack of respect for the marriage union? When interacting with your married friends, are you showing the most attention to your friend's husband? Do you seek private conversation with him? Do you call your friends' husband to plan events? Do you seek out married men on social media? Do you continually come up with things which we need *"the husband's help"* (i.e. change a light bulb)? Do you show up at your friend's house when she's not home and end up spending time with her husband? Are you confiding in a married man and sharing your heart with him? If the answer to any of these questions is yes, then I would highly question what's happening in your heart. In today's world, more than half of marriages will suffer through an affair. Most affairs begin with friendship, a counseling situation, or a work relationship. The most likely person to be an affair partner is a close friend of the opposite sex. But, isn't our spouse supposed to be our best friend?

Affairs begin with dissatisfaction in the mind. Too many marriages have been destroyed by men who transfer their desires to a young air-brushed fantasy on-line, in a magazine, or in sleazy movies. When a mind is focused on physical perfection, will an aging bride ever satisfy? Too many marriages have also been destroyed by a woman who is not satisfied with her position in the home, expecting her husband to give in to her control. Decisions become one-sided. When respect is lost for a husband who cannot fill a need for satisfaction that only God can fill, she turns her focus outside the relationship. The illusion is that the grass is always greener on the other side; the truth is that the grass is only green on the side that is watered.

We need to water our side of the fence. Your marriage is like a garden to water, protect, nurture, and cherish. Keep the weeds and the dogs out! Guard the sanctity of your marriage. Too many of us live with the destruction of divorce. Before we become reckless, shall we be prudent? If God gives you someone, why would you not cherish them?

Be wise. Be careful. Be prudent.

"The foolishness of a man twists his way,
And his heart frets against the Lord."
~Proverbs 19:3

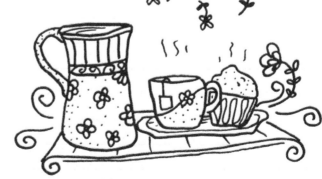

CREATIVE JOURNALING

Today's Date: _____

In Proverbs **19,** which verse pops out to you? How does that verse apply to your world today? Journal honestly about your respect to the sanctity of marriage, whether it is yours, or your friends or relatives marriages;

_____
_____
_____
_____
_____
_____
_____
_____
_____
_____
_____
_____
_____
_____
_____
_____
_____
_____
_____
_____
_____
_____
_____
_____
_____
_____
_____
_____
_____
_____
_____
_____

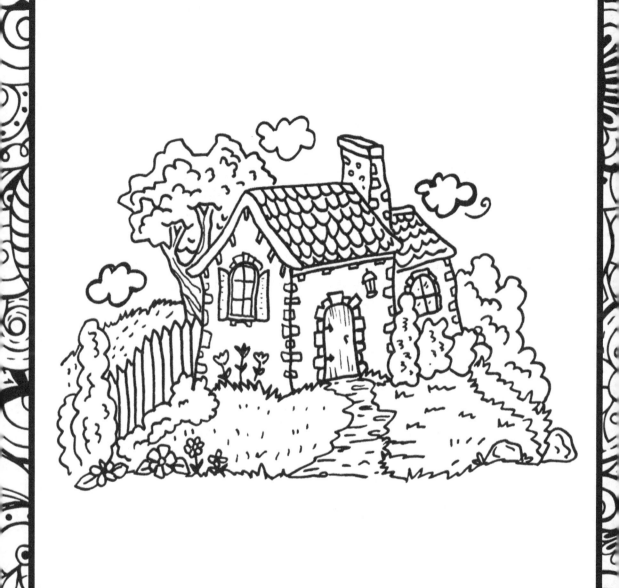

"A foolish child is a calamity to a father;
a quarrelsome wife is as annoying
as constant dripping."
~Proverbs 19:13

Day 20 ~ Proverbs 20

"False weights and unequal measures—
the Lord detests double standards of every kind."
~Proverbs **20:10** (NLT)

How often we cheat at the little things. We tend to believe that God only admonishes the "big" sins and that the little blunders don't count. Are you honest when the store clerk gives you too much change, or do you keep the overage? Do you pay back that quarter you borrowed, or do you dismiss such a small amount of money? What about that pen you accidentally kept after signing the receipt? Do you walk all the way back to return it?

"The buyer haggles over the price, saying, "It's worthless,"
then brags about getting a bargain!"
~Proverbs **20:14** (NLT)

Some people hate to negotiate. Some of it is sheer personality, but mostly, negotiating is an indication that one of the parties is attempting to get something for nothing. Either the seller has inflated the price to portray something more than it is worth, or the buyer (as in the Proverb) is casting doubt on the quality in order to pay less than the actual worth. The purchase is actually deceptive theft.

"Stolen bread tastes sweet,
but it turns to gravel in the mouth."
~Proverbs **20:17** (NLT)

Showing a double standard is all too common in our relationships as well as our finances. The same irritations we have toward others are often times overlooked in ourselves. Overlooking a sin in one person (me!) but having higher expectations by condemning the same sin in another is a double standard. A lot of times our insecurities show in the perfection we portray to the outside world. We Christians sometimes tend to wear "masks" to hide our imperfections. We are fearful of rejection by our peers if we show our faults. As long as we are accepting of others, perhaps God will allow us to hide for a while. But, when we show impatience and contempt for others in the same characteristics which we hide beneath our own mask, we are living on an imbalanced scale. Wearing a mask is living a lie.

"The Lord detests double standards;
he is not pleased by dishonest scales."
~Proverbs **20:23** (NLT)

Today's chapter contains several verses pertaining to cheating or theft. I believe a lot of the Proverbs are spoken to those who already follow God, not the heathens. Why would Christians need to be reminded of basic honesty? Because, we are still working out our salvation (Philippians **2:12-16**). We live in a fallen world, born with a nature of sin. This is why we have been saved by grace. Jesus paid the debt for our sin for none of us are able to fulfill the law on our own.

"Let nothing be done through selfish ambition or conceit, but in lowliness of mind let each esteem others better than himself. Let each of you look out not only for his own interests, but also for the interests of others."
~Philippians **2:3-4**

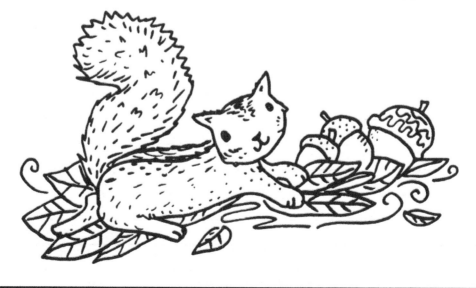

CREATIVE JOURNALING

Today's Date: _____

In Proverbs 20, which verse pops out to you? How does that verse apply to your world today? Were there times you gave into temptation to take shortcuts? What were your consequences?

_____
_____
_____
_____
_____
_____
_____
_____
_____
_____
_____
_____
_____
_____
_____
_____
_____
_____
_____
_____
_____
_____
_____
_____
_____
_____
_____

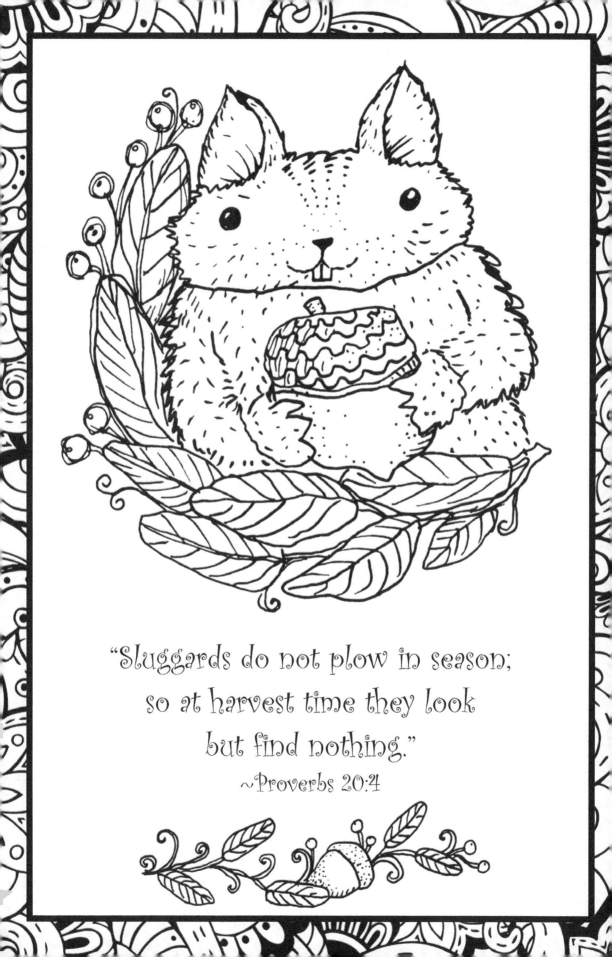

"Sluggards do not plow in season;
so at harvest time they look
but find nothing."
~Proverbs 20:4

Day 21 ~ Proverbs 21

*"It is better to dwell in a corner of the housetop,
than with a brawling woman in a wide house."*
~Proverbs **21:9** (KJV)

This verse always seems humorous. I can just envision the big burly man hanging on to the corner of the roof while the little woman is inside behaving as if she were in a bar fight! The context of the verse is usually relayed as a husband who cannot handle his contentious wife. Many a sermon on the wife's submission has referred to this verse.

I believe there is a much deeper meaning. When the context is looked at through the time period which it was written, we get a better understanding of the meaning. In Eastern countries, the roofs were flat and used as an extra gathering space. Even today, people often sleep on the rooftops due to the heat. The rooftops were often used as we use our patios or balconies. Meetings and gatherings were held on the rooftops to ensure privacy. People used the rooftops as a quiet retreat and for prayer. Acts **10:9** says, *"...Peter went up on the housetop to pray, about the sixth hour."*

In those days, a wide house indicated either a house of society or a house large enough for more than one family to live in. It was common practice for a couple to live with the parents from the beginning of their marriage. My first thought is that too many cooks in the same kitchen are recipes for a brawl. If a woman is angry or bitter, she will have plenty of people around to create drama.

Why would he want to live on the corner? Usually the roof was as wide as the house itself. In the corner, he is subject to the elements of weather. Wind will be stronger at the corners. The danger of falling off would be greater. This would indicate that the husband would rather live without comfort than to put up with his wife's contentious nagging. This would seem to be an admonition to women. And it is true, we are all guilty of nagging every once in a while.

"Better to dwell in the wilderness,
Than with a contentious and angry woman."
~Proverbs 21:19

Would the writer hint to an admonition to the husband as well? Isn't the husband to be the head of the household? If he were leading a house full of love he would have no need to live on the corner. How do we counteract contention? What is the best way to produce peace? 1st John 4:7-8 says; *"Beloved, let us love one another, for love is of God; and everyone who loves is born of God and knows God. He who does not love does not know God, for God is love."* We dispel hatred and anger with love. The book of Ephesians teaches us how to walk in love. Ephesians 2:14 says; *"For He Himself is our peace, who has made both one, and has broken down the middle wall of separation..."* We find Jesus' peace through forgiveness, being kind to one another, and loving our spouse as taught in the 4th and 5th chapters.

Finally, in the last chapter, Ephesians 6:12 (NIV), we are told, *"For our struggle is not against flesh and blood, but against the rulers, against the authorities, against the powers of this dark world and against the spiritual forces of evil in the heavenly realms."* Since our spouse is not our enemy, how do we fight through this struggle? With prayer: *"And pray in the Spirit on all occasions with all kinds of prayers and requests. With this in mind, be alert and always keep on praying for all the Lord's people."* Ephesians 6:18 (NIV).

Maybe the husband should go to the rooftop and seek God in prayer for his household? And the wives need to follow...

The family that prays together...stays together...

CREATIVE JOURNALING

Today's Date: _____

In Proverbs **21**, which verse pops out to you? How does that verse apply to your world today? Have you prayed for and with your family today?

_____

_____

_____

_____

_____

_____

_____

_____

_____

_____

_____

_____

_____

_____

_____

_____

_____

_____

_____

_____

_____

_____

_____

_____

_____

_____

_____

_____

_____

_____

_____

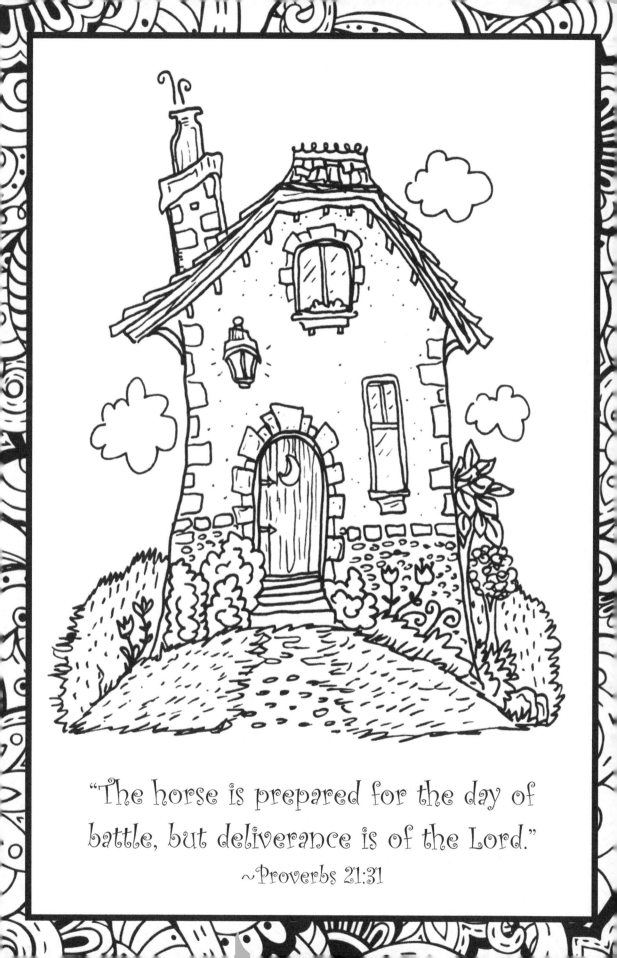

"The horse is prepared for the day of battle, but deliverance is of the Lord."
~Proverbs 21:31

Day 22 ~ Proverbs 22

"Train up a child in the way he should go,
And when he is old he will not depart from it." ~Proverbs **22:6**

Most people equate the sixth verse in Proverbs **22** with discipline, or even with finances. But I believe God had much more in mind when he gave Solomon this inspiration. *Train up* in the Hebrew, חנך, means to initiate, or to instruct a child. *The way he should go* indicates the path, future calling, or station in life that the child should follow. *The way he should go* also indicates the character traits and natural inclination of his/her temperament that form the qualifications for his/her particular path.

A study of the different temperaments provides very helpful tools for all our relationships. We begin to understand how different we were created and how God uses those differences to bind us together. When we understand the individual qualities of our children, we are able to give them the freedom to grow in their *own* character. How often do parents vicariously live their lives through their children? When my own children were young, nowhere did I see this phenomenon more than in the sports arena. My boys' soccer coach eventually enforced a rule that no one on the sideline was allowed to shout at any of the players. Some of those parents were more out of control than the soccer ball! When you try to force your own life on another, we all lose.

"A good name is to be chosen rather than great riches,
Loving favor rather than silver and gold." ~Proverbs **22:1**

Every child is created in God's image. No one is perfect, but God created everyone with talents and qualities that make each person valuable. 1st Corinthians **12** teaches we are all different, yet we are all valuable and each diverse part is needed for the body to function properly. A parent's biggest defeat is when a child is forced to become a person they were not created to be. Ephesians 6:4 says, *"And you, fathers, do not provoke your children to wrath, but bring them up in the training and admonition of the Lord."* We must ask ourselves: Do I bring my children up in the admonition (council or instruction) of the Lord or of my own desire for who I want them to become?

"Do you see a man who excels in his work?
  He will stand before kings;
He will not stand before unknown men." ~Proverbs 22:29

By bringing up a child in our own image, we are in essence saying we love ourselves and not the child. When we build up the characteristics of the child's own DNA, he/she will reflect the image of God. The child's talents will be multiplied (Matthew 25:20) when they function in the natural abilities he/she was born. You can't fit a round peg in a square hole. If a child is right-brained wired for creativity he/she will not flourish in a left-brained analytical arena, and vise-verse. A parent's relationship will suffer if the child who was born to paint murals or create music is coerced into a corporate profession. And likewise, if the child loves numbers and books, he may not be the NFL football player you desire. Will you love them anyway?

"Everybody is a genius. But if you judge a fish by its ability to climb a tree, it will live its whole life believing that it is stupid." ~Amos E. Dolbear of Tufts, a prominent physicist and inventor.

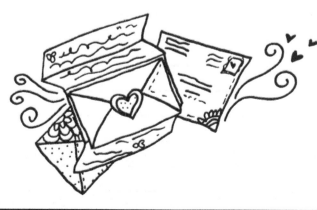

CREATIVE JOURNALING

Today's Date: _____

In Proverbs **22,** which verse pops out to you? How does that verse apply to your world today? Are you allowing those around you to have the freedom to live as the people God created them to be? How can you help others develop their own talents?

_____
_____
_____
_____
_____
_____
_____
_____
_____
_____
_____
_____
_____
_____
_____
_____
_____
_____
_____
_____
_____
_____
_____
_____
_____

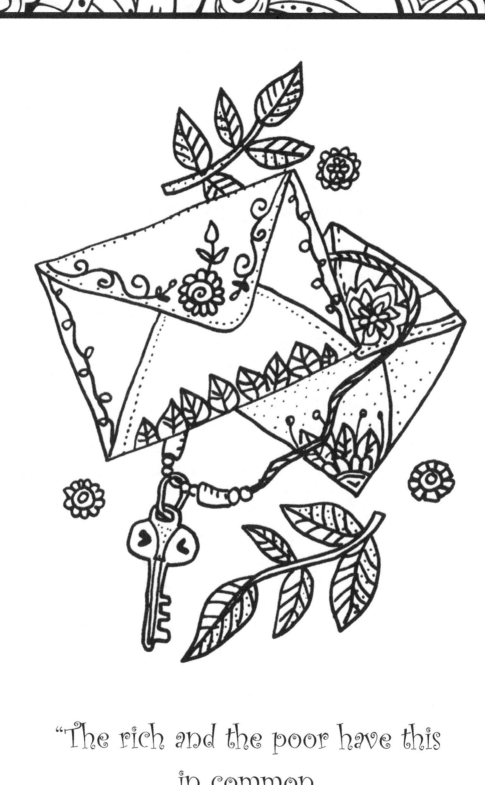

"The rich and the poor have this
in common,
the LORD is the maker of them all."
~Proverbs 22:2

Day 23 ~ Proverbs 23

"They have struck me, but I was not hurt; they have beaten me, but I did not feel it. When shall I awake, that I may seek another drink?" ~Proverbs **23:35** (TLB)

The last six verses of today's Proverb gives a vivid description of a drunkard. I believe that young youth would never take the first drink if technology ever advances to show a futuristic video of him or her plastered and hammered. Drunkards are incapable of seeing how ridiculous they look.

Alcohol is a natural preservative. Medical research has shown that alcohol is good for you, but only in moderation (less than one drink a day). It's said that alcohol is both a tonic and a poison depending on the dose. According to medical research, small amounts (less than a glass a day) has been proven to benefit the heart, circulatory system, blood clotting, and helps protect against type **2** diabetes and gallstones. On the other hand, heavy drinking can damage the liver and heart, harm unborn babies, and is a major contributor to depression and violence (please research the benefits and dangers for yourself). Alcohol is the most commonly used addictive substance in the U.S. One in every **12** adults, or **17.6** million people, suffer from alcohol abuse or dependence. According to the National Highway Traffic Safety Administration (NHTSA), **31%** of all traffic deaths in **2013** in the United States (latest figures available), died in drunk driving crashes, making it the fourth leading preventable cause of death in the United States. Alcoholism not only destroys relationships, it destroys lives.

I don't want today's devotional to be negative. Alcohol in and of itself is not evil, just as money is not evil. What we do with the thing is what makes it evil. Alcohol can be used for good purposes, just as money can be used positively. The Apostle Paul stated in 1st Timothy 5:23, *"No longer drink only water, but use a little wine for your stomach's sake and your frequent infirmities."* Jesus' first miracle was turning the water into wine: *"And he said to him, "Every man at the beginning sets out the good wine, and when the guests have well drunk, then the inferior. You have kept the good wine until now!"* John 2:10. I've heard both arguments for and against the strength of the fermentation of the wine. I don't believe it matters whether you believe it was fermented grapes or common juice, the principle is the same. It's about self-control.

"Do not mix with winebibbers, or with gluttonous eaters of meat; for the drunkard and the glutton will come to poverty, and drowsiness will clothe a man with rags."
~Proverbs **23:20-21**

A thorough reading of the Proverbs shows Solomon warned against habits, addictions, and sin in every area. I find it interesting that in most places in the bible, a drunkard is grouped with a glutton. Deuteronomy **21:19-21** groups the two together. 1st Corinthians **6:9-11** & Galatians **5:20-22** says gluttons will not inherit the Kingdom of God. Proverbs **28:7** says, *"Whoever keeps the law is a discerning son, but a companion of gluttons shames his father."* I also find it interesting and rather hypocritical that a lot of people I know who preach against drinking...are gluttons. The level of self-control you exercise makes all the difference in the outcome in *every* area of your life.

Remember Proverbs **16:18**? *"Pride goes before destruction, and a haughty spirit before a fall."* If you think you may be struggling with an addiction or a hang-up; whether it is alcohol, drugs, food, anger, co-dependency, etc., please don't be too proud to seek help. Pray. Contact a trusted pastor, friend, or seek out a local Celebrate Recovery™ or another biblical based program. Not only will your life benefit, but so will those closest to you!

CREATIVE JOURNALING

Today's Date: _____

In Proverbs **23,** which verse pops out to you? How does that verse apply to your world today? Journal about any areas in your life that have become unmanageable:

_____

_____

_____

_____

_____

_____

_____

_____

_____

_____

_____

_____

_____

_____

_____

_____

_____

_____

_____

_____

_____

_____

_____

_____

_____

_____

_____

_____

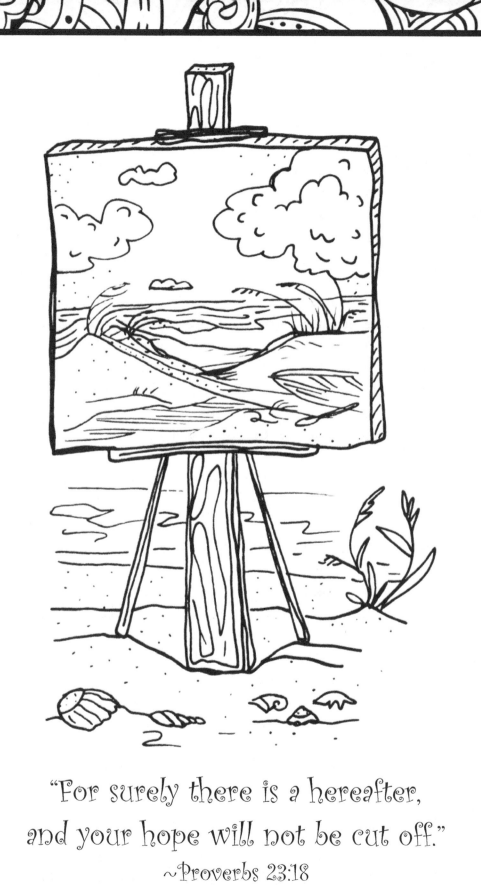

"For surely there is a hereafter,
and your hope will not be cut off."
~Proverbs 23:18

Day 24 ~ Proverbs 24

"Rescue those who are unjustly sentenced to die;
save them as they stagger to their death.
Don't excuse yourself by saying, "Look, we didn't know."
For God understands all hearts, and he sees you.
He who guards your soul knows you knew.
He will repay all people as their actions deserve."
~Proverbs **24:11–12** (TLB)

Every time I read this verse my heart aches for the innocent: the unborn, the euthanized, the Holocaust, genocide in Africa, etc. Some of these instances have become political hot spots. While we are not addressing political issues, we *are* addressing biblical issues. Life is imperative to God. He is our creator. He not only weeps over our physical death, He weeps over our relational death, for our heart.

These verses deal with the crime of negligence. James **2:17** says, "*Therefore, to him who knows to do good and does not do it, to him it is sin.*" We are instructed by God to walk in righteousness. But what does that look like? Does walking in righteousness only reflect our own behavior? We don't get drunk, we don't smoke, we don't get high, and we don't cuss like a Sailor. But, are we justified by the outside? Jesus said in Luke **16:15**, "*And He said to them, "You are those who justify yourselves before men, but God knows your hearts. For what is highly esteemed among men is an abomination in the sight of God.*" If God knows our hearts, He knows that when we sit silently we consent to immorality, to sin. What is immorality? It is defined as: *transgressing accepted moral rules or principles of right conduct or the distinction between right and wrong and that which is ethical; being corrupt.* God looks at our heart.

"But those who rebuke the wicked will have delight,
And a good blessing will come upon them." ~Proverbs **24:25**

One of the most used verses for blame-shifting our responsibility is Proverbs 26:17: *"He who passes by and meddles in a quarrel not his own is like one who takes a dog by the ears."* No one wants to be the little old town busy-body lady that sticks her nose into everybody's business, and then turns around and gossips. But, on the other extreme, to ignore injustice only encourages anarchy. A child who is allowed to bully others at a young age will grow up to cause harm to society. God's heart is for the underdog. Jesus died for those who could not escape from their own sin...all of us.

The difference is Love. Love is not walking in anger, controlling others, or in being unkind. And yet, Love is definitely not silent. Proverbs 27:6 says, *"Faithful are the wounds of a friend, but the kisses of an enemy are deceitful."* Love desires the best for us. When we stand up for injustice, not only are we helping the life of the innocent, but we are saving the life of the offender. James puts it this way in 5:19 -20, *"Brethren, if anyone among you wanders from the truth, and someone turns him back, let him know that he who turns a sinner from the error of his way will save a soul from death and cover a multitude of sins."* Do we fear repercussions of others? Take to heart the words in 1st John 4:18, *"There is no fear in love..."*

Who has the Lord called you to *"rescue"* today?

"Do not fret because of evildoers,
Nor be envious of the wicked;
For there will be no prospect for the evil man;
The lamp of the wicked will be put out."
~Proverbs 24:19-20

CREATIVE JOURNALING

Today's Date: _____

In Proverbs **24,** which verse pops out to you? How does that verse apply to your world today? Was there a time in your life in which someone defended you against an injustice? Have you defended others?

_____
_____
_____
_____
_____
_____
_____
_____
_____
_____
_____
_____
_____
_____
_____
_____
_____
_____
_____
_____
_____
_____
_____
_____
_____
_____
_____
_____

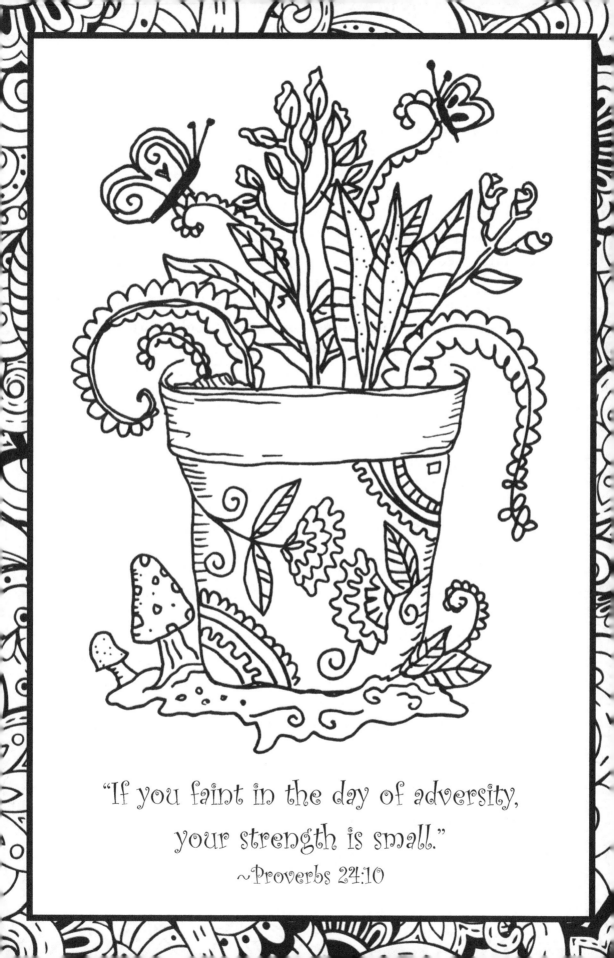

"If you faint in the day of adversity,
your strength is small."
~Proverbs 24:10

Day 25 ~ Proverbs 25

"Remove the dross from the silver,
and out comes material for the silversmith..."
~Proverbs **25:4** (NIV)

I love the analogy of the Refiner! A refiner will heat the gold or silver to a temperature so hot that all the impurities (past hurts, bitterness selfishness, envy, etc.) are burned away. The refiner only starts the cooling process when he is able to see His own reflection (forgiveness, peace, joy, etc.) in the liquid. You see, when the Lord refines us, he not only burns out the dirt in our life he also changes our molecules, our core, and our thinking process. When we have been refined, we begin to see ourselves as the Lord does; beautiful, pure, and worthy of the sacrifice He gave long before we were born.

It took me most of my life, a lot of soul-searching, and a ton of prayers to begin to see myself the way the Lord sees me. I, like most people, grew up with an inaccurate belief system of what makes a person acceptable. There has been so much talk the past couple of decades about the "blame it on my childhood" syndrome that it's become a crutch and excuse for everything wrong in life. Blame-shifting does not heal. I believe while it is very true your past experiences can determine your outlook today (and need to be dealt with); your past experiences, nor that which others believe from your past, do not dictate who you are in Christ. According to God's word (see Deuteronomy **24:16** & 2 Kings **14:5-7**) we are responsible for ourselves...and our worth is based on God's opinion, not man's opinion. When I stopped trying to live up to the world's (parents, family, church, friends) unattainable standards, and began to focus on the things the Lord said about me: that I'm restored, completely accepted, and cherished; then I found the peace, security, and comfort that can only come from God.

I don't get discouraged when God corrects my patterns of thought. Though sometimes his correction humbles us, he is growing our character. For unlike our earthly fathers, His correction is unselfish and always for our good, in our best interest, and given in love. It takes being *refined* before we can fully appreciate just how much the Lord loves us and how valued we are, thereby freeing us to love others.

"Remove wicked officials from the king's presence,
and his throne will be established through righteousness."
~Proverbs **25:5** (NIV)

God not only refines our sin nature and our thought process, he refines our social life. **2**nd Peter **2:20** says, *"If they have escaped the corruption of the world by knowing our Lord and Savior Jesus Christ and are again entangled in it and are overcome, they are worse off at the end than they were at the beginning."* (NIV) Birds of a feather flock together. Removing wicked people from our inner circle not only applies to the kings in Solomon's day, it applies to us today. Grace enables us to love people without following in their sin. Jesus gave us examples through his friendships. Though Jesus taught and ministered to thousands of evil people, he did not invite them into his inner circle, (except for Judas, whom Jesus knew to be evil, that God's plan for his death be fulfilled). Of the twelve disciples, he was even closer to three; Peter, James, and John. Jesus loved, forgave, and restored the least of the least, he never negated sin. He said in John **5:14**, *"See, you have been made well. Sin no more, lest a worse thing come upon you."* We will live without the drama of destructive relationships if we surround ourselves with other believers who build us up and point us to Christ.

Spend time in prayer today asking the Lord to lead you in every relationship.

CREATIVE JOURNALING

Today's Date: _____

In Proverbs 25, which verse pops out to you? How does that verse apply to your world today? What negative thoughts do you have about yourself? What does God believe about you? Do your thoughts line up with God's word?

_____
_____
_____
_____
_____
_____
_____
_____
_____
_____
_____
_____
_____
_____
_____
_____
_____
_____
_____
_____
_____
_____
_____
_____
_____
_____
_____
_____

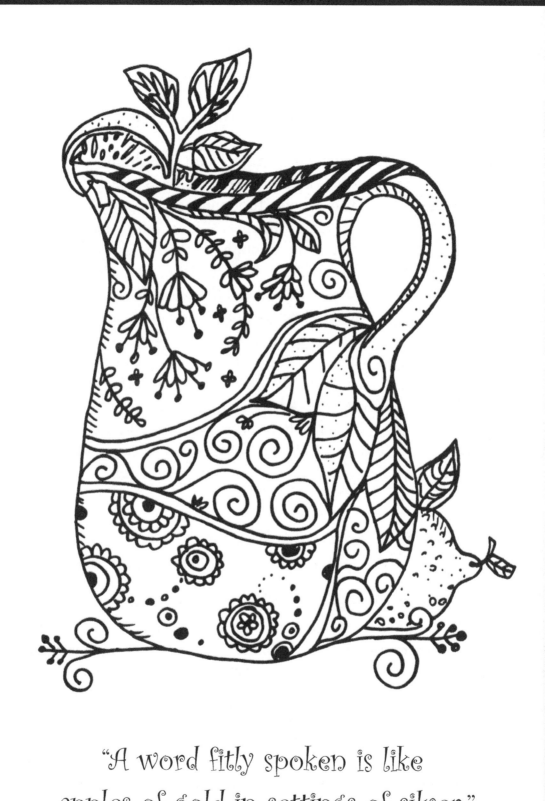

"A word fitly spoken is like
apples of gold in settings of silver."
~Proverbs 25:11

Day 26 ~ Proverbs 26

"As a dog returns to his own vomit,
So a fool repeats his folly." ~Proverbs **26:11**

I could leave any discussion of this chapter right here. Is there any further explanation needed? The visual should be enough to make anyone stop their foolishness and turn down a straight path! For some people, especially men, simply changing a baby's diaper is enough to churn a stomach, let alone vomit. But, return to our folly we do...

The Apostle Paul very frustratingly admonishes in the 7th chapter of Romans how our sin nature drags us back into doing the things we don't want to do. Verse **15** says, *"For what I am doing, I do not understand. For what I will to do, that I do not practice; but what I hate, that I do."* And, verse **19**, *"For the good that I will to do, I do not do; but the evil I will not to do, that I practice."* Why do we tend to regress back into our own stupidity? Do you ever get discouraged making the same mistakes over again?

"Do you see a man wise in his own eyes?
There is more hope for a fool than for him." ~Proverbs **26:12**

Most mountain climber fatalities take place on the descent, not the ascent. I found that statistic a bit odd until I understood the technique. Climbers put an enormous amount of technical care in the climb. The adrenaline rushes with the will of the soul to reach the top. Once on the top of the mountain, the drive settles down. Without a new goal, we flounder around in arrogant nothingness, gloating in our accomplishment. We tend to get lethargic and lazy. We relax just a little too much. Our pride and arrogance has consumed our walk, for now we can accomplish anything. That's when carelessness sets in and the foot slips...

We are all works in progress. Humility admits that we are fragile beings in need. Every time we as Christians fall, we hurt the Gospel more than those who were never believers. We fall when we take our eyes off of the Lord, focusing on our own accomplishments. I realized years ago that my own independence, while quite an asset most of the time, can quite easily turn into pride and self-sufficiency. The second we disregard the helping hand of the Lord, we fall prey to evil. Each time we fall, the vomit sours over again. 2nd Peter 2:21-22 reiterates Solomon's Proverb: *"For it would have been better for them not to have known the way of righteousness, than having known it, to turn from the holy commandment delivered to them. But it has happened to them according to the true proverb: "A dog returns to his own vomit," and, "a sow, having washed, to her wallowing in the mire."* Yuk!

How do we keep from being the fool? Paul tells us in Romans 7:25: *"Thank God! The answer is in Jesus Christ our Lord. So you see how it is: In my mind I really want to obey God's law, but because of my sinful nature I am a slave to sin."* But we do have hope! Jesus made sure anyone who believes and trusts in Him would have God's help through the Holy Spirit: *"But the Helper, the Holy Spirit, whom the Father will send in My name, He will teach you all things, and bring to your remembrance all things that I said to you. Peace I leave with you, My peace I give to you; not as the world gives do I give to you. Let not your heart be troubled, neither let it be afraid."* John 14:26-27

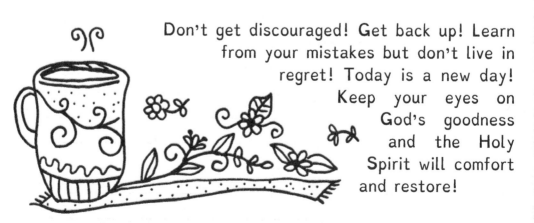

Don't get discouraged! Get back up! Learn from your mistakes but don't live in regret! Today is a new day! Keep your eyes on God's goodness and the Holy Spirit will comfort and restore!

CREATIVE JOURNALING

Today's Date: _____

In Proverbs 26, which verse pops out to you? How does that verse apply to your world today? What mistakes and habits are you repeating from your past?

_____
_____
_____
_____
_____
_____
_____
_____
_____
_____
_____
_____
_____
_____
_____
_____
_____
_____
_____
_____
_____
_____
_____
_____
_____
_____
_____
_____

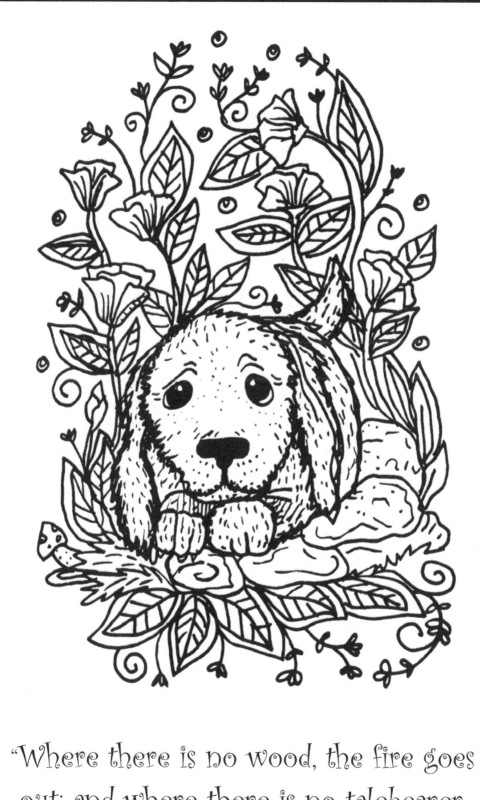

"Where there is no wood, the fire goes out; and where there is no talebearer, strife ceases." ~Proverbs 26:20

Day 27 ~ Proverbs 27

*"Do not boast about tomorrow,
for you do not know what a day may bring."* ~**Proverbs 27:1**

It is said the only constant in life is change. I don't believe change in and of itself is neither good nor bad. It just is. The insecure and fearful soul will fight change. The stubborn and controlling soul will fight change. But sometimes...the very tired soul will grow weary of change.

Life can crush our spirit. With change, God can refresh our circumstances...and our spirit. With each birth or death a new era is born. With each change a new hope is secured.

We know the birth of one baby will change the whole dynamics of a family...even to the extended family. We can't help but love the innocent. Our whole attention is focused on caring for and nurturing the new little life. We build bigger houses and rearrange our schedules to accommodate our new little addition. Some people experience the same changes with the addition of a pet! Yesterday, the house was quiet...today it is full of noise. We look into the face of the innocent and our spirits rise with the hope of a new future.

Yet, since we don't miss what we don't know, if that person or relationship was never there, we would never experience the love. But, when we love what we know, and that love is ripped from us, our world is full of empty holes. Just as a family changes with a birth, the death of one person will change the whole dynamics of that family...even to the extended family. With one phone call, one hospital visit, just one person gone, our tomorrows feel the void of that loved one. Our holidays change, our birthdays change, even our phone calls and emails change. How different would we have treated that person who is now gone had we known the difference a day would bring?

As I sit here writing, hurricane Matthew is wreaking havoc through the Atlantic. When we arrange our life, do we consider how even a natural disaster can change our whole future? In Luke 6:38 Jesus said, *"Give, and it will be given to you."* Most commentaries link Proverbs 27:1 with Matthew 6:34, Luke 12:13-34, and James 4:13-17. Of those listed, I love the analogy Jesus gave of the man who built bigger barns to hold all of his belongings. That very night, his life was snuffed out. I wonder if he would have behaved differently if he understood that a day would end his future plans. Would he have built bigger barns, or given his hoards away? Would he have used his hoards to bless others, or would he have set up monuments in his name? The parable brings back memories of the 2009 TV show, *Hoarders.* Unfortunately, the experts of today have labeled the condition as a mental illness, whereas God labeled it greed...sin. In Jesus' parable, the hoarder left this world leaving his hoarded belongings behind. We all do. Job 1:21 says, *"Naked I came from my mother's womb, and naked shall I return there."*

I just wonder if the world would be a better place if everyone grasped the concept of the flower of Matthew 6:30, *"Now if God so clothes the grass of the field, which today is, and tomorrow is thrown into the oven, will He not much more clothe you, O you of little faith?"* Would our insecurities of change subside? Would our stranglehold of the material loosen? Would we relax and quit boasting or worrying about tomorrow?

Embrace the here and now. Let go of the past. Give God the future. For we never know what a day may bring...

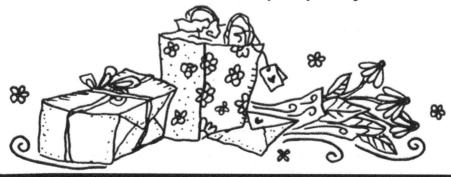

CREATIVE JOURNALING

Today's Date: _____

In Proverbs 27, which verse pops out to you? How does that verse apply to your world today? Journal how you can embrace change and not cling to relationships or material possessions:

_____

_____

_____

_____

_____

_____

_____

_____

_____

_____

_____

_____

_____

_____

_____

_____

_____

_____

_____

_____

_____

_____

_____

_____

_____

_____

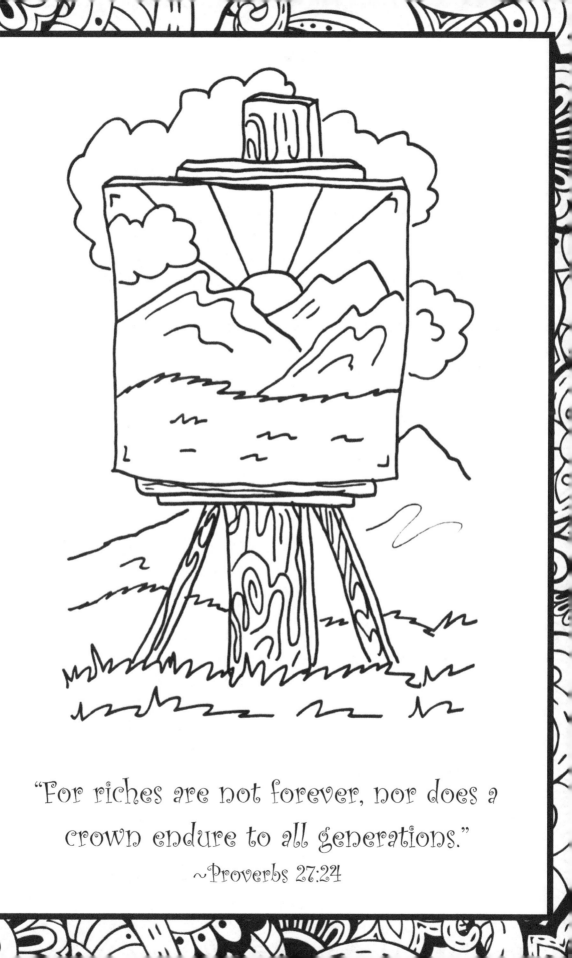

"For riches are not forever, nor does a crown endure to all generations."
~Proverbs 27:24

Day 28 ~ Proverbs 28

*"He who tills his land will have plenty of bread,
But he who follows frivolity will have poverty enough!"*
                                        ~Proverbs 28:19

What kind of friends do we keep? Do they lift us up or drag us down? Do we interpret *lifting up* as making one happy and encouraging a continual party? Or do our friends encourage us to strive for the best in ourselves and develop Godly goals? The friends we keep help develop our character and our future. The words that fill our ears affect our thought patterns. When we follow friends who are frivolous and live in a continual party mode, we begin to slip into those same patterns. After all, how hard is it to work a full week while receiving continual message requests to skip off to the mall, salon, or the beach? We put our job, as well as any chance of advancement, at risk of collapse. We ultimately find ourselves in poverty.

I like how the NIV puts the second half; *"But the one who chases fantasies will have his fill of poverty."* This version is a great analogy of the *get rich* schemes of today. Advertisers take advantage of lazy people (who in their greed want something for nothing) by promising high returns for very little input, whereas the scheme rarely brings profit for the participant. Many marriages have been wrecked from a spouse who secretly spent savings on get rich Money Trading and Wall Street ventures. Anything hidden from your spouse is not of God, for God is light. If you don't trust the Lord to be your provider, your faith is in the temporal. If you believe your worth is established in wealth, you will end up chasing fantasies.

*"Better is the poor who walks in his integrity
Than one perverse in his ways, though he be rich."*
                                        ~Proverbs 28:6

Money in and of itself is not the enemy. However, the love of the world's money for our own pleasure is where destruction lies. To prosper in earthly wealth is not the satisfying prosperity God has to offer. As with everything else, God looks at the heart. If your heart is clouded with unforgiveness and selfishness, you will not have the peace and joy of His prosperity. God desires his children to have *all* he has to offer. Wealth is already his. He *created* the earth! But *how* we obtain our material possessions and the friends we keep determines the quality of our heart. When we promote ourselves by befriending the rich, or that popular friend, for our own benefit, we are living in self-centeredness without integrity. James 2:5-6 says, *"Listen, my beloved brethren: Has God not chosen the poor of this world to be rich in faith and heirs of the kingdom which He promised to those who love Him? But you have dishonored the poor man. Do not the rich oppress you and drag you into the courts?"* Are these the kind of friends you want? But, to have friends of integrity, you must have integrity. The best way to check your heart is to look at how you treat others on your way up that ladder. What kind of prosperity do you desire? Do you desire the world's wealth or to prosper in all that God has for you?

"Whoever gives to the poor will lack nothing,
    but those who close their eyes to poverty will be cursed."
                                                    ~Proverbs 28:27

The concept of giving to others so God can give to us is all too foreign. Acts 20:35 says, *"It is more blessed to give than to receive."* To be rich with God's wealth is a blessing, to be rich with that which we did not earn righteously is a curse. An old saying that is proven trusted and true: "If you take care of the things of God, He will take care of you." This comes from Psalm 37:4, *"Delight yourself also in the Lord, and He shall give you the desires of your heart."* Do you trust Him to provide? Will you be satisfied with the Lord's provision?

In His hand is the only place true contentment is found.

CREATIVE JOURNALING

Today's Date: _____

In Proverbs 28, which verse pops out to you? How does that verse apply to your world today? Do you see God's wealth in your life? Or, do you see the world's wealth?

_____
_____
_____
_____
_____
_____
_____
_____
_____
_____
_____
_____
_____
_____
_____
_____
_____
_____
_____
_____
_____
_____
_____
_____
_____
_____
_____
_____

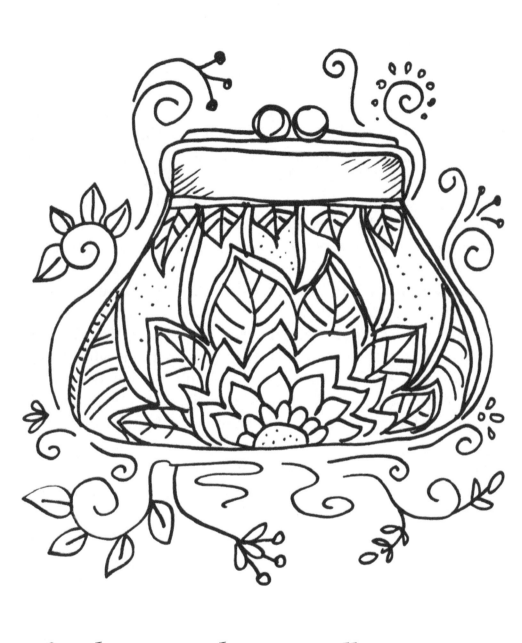

"He who covers his sins will not prosper,
but whoever confesses and
forsakes them will have mercy."
~Proverbs 28:13

Day 29 ~ Proverbs 29

"By transgression an evil man is snared,
But the righteous sings and rejoices." ~Proverbs **29:6**

A snare is a trap used to capture animals. The animal is usually badly hurt or killed when caught in the hunter's snare. Animals are driven by instinct and fleshly desires. The hunter will tempt the animal into the lair with bait that is craved by that particular animal. The animal, not knowing its demise, follows its desire to satisfy its flesh, only to find death in the offing.

Transgression means to violate a law, to sin. An evil man, or woman, is a person without God's spirit. Someone who does not know God cannot be expected to adhere to the same standard of righteousness. This is the person who has no desire to seek God or His goodness. This person lives in the desires of the world and what will satisfy the flesh, or what *feels* good. Unrealized sin is the snare that leads to death.

"Do not love the world or the things in the world. If anyone loves the world, the love of the Father is not in him. For all that is in the world—the lust of the flesh, the lust of the eyes, and the pride of life—is not of the Father but is of the world. And the world is passing away, and the lust of it; but he who does the will of God abides forever." ~**1**st John **2:15–17**

What is it that snares us? Like the animal heading into the lair, what draws someone without God's guidance? Left on our own, we seek to fill our stomachs with wealth, position, entertainment, etc. A snare can be anything that keeps you from seeking the Lord. Busyness can be a snare. How can we develop a close relationship with God if we are too busy to read His word? Our friends can be a snare. Do they encourage us to seek God's path or on the road of fun or negativity? What is your daily snare?

"The fear of man brings a snare,
But whoever trusts in the Lord shall be safe." ~Proverbs **29:25**

Fear is a devastating snare. When we fear people, we become people-pleasers instead of God-pleasers. How can we recognize when we fear people? Observe where your desires lay. Do you live in the insecurity of waking up without friends? Do you long for the approval and applause of people, or are you satisfied without receiving credit for your deeds? Do you seek God's approval? Do you fear ridicule from people? Do you fear persecution or death? 1st John **4:18** says, *"There is no fear in love; but perfect love casts out fear, because fear involves torment. But he who fears has not been made perfect in love."* Real love is free of fear.

Worry is a snare that pulls us away from the Lord. When we fear people, our comfort, or the future, we live in continual worry from not trusting in God's provision. Do we not trust that the creator of the universe is capable of taking care of all our little details in life? Remember John **3:16**? *"For God so loved the world that He gave His only begotten Son, that whoever believes in Him should not perish but have everlasting life."* If God went to that much trouble and sacrifice for us, why would we not trust Him?

When we are living with a conscience free of habitual sin, we experience His peace. When we trust in God for our daily lives, we have no fear. This freedom and peace in God's righteousness and love brings deep joy. When joy abounds, our souls overflow with rejoicing which is expressed in joyous songs.

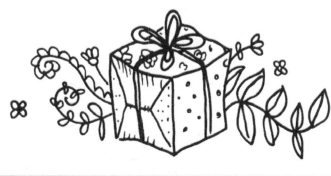

CREATIVE JOURNALING

Today's Date: _____

In Proverbs 29, which verse pops out to you? How does that verse apply to your world today? Are you snared by fear? Journal the cause of your fears:

_____
_____
_____
_____
_____
_____
_____
_____
_____
_____
_____
_____
_____
_____
_____
_____
_____
_____
_____
_____
_____
_____
_____
_____
_____
_____
_____
_____

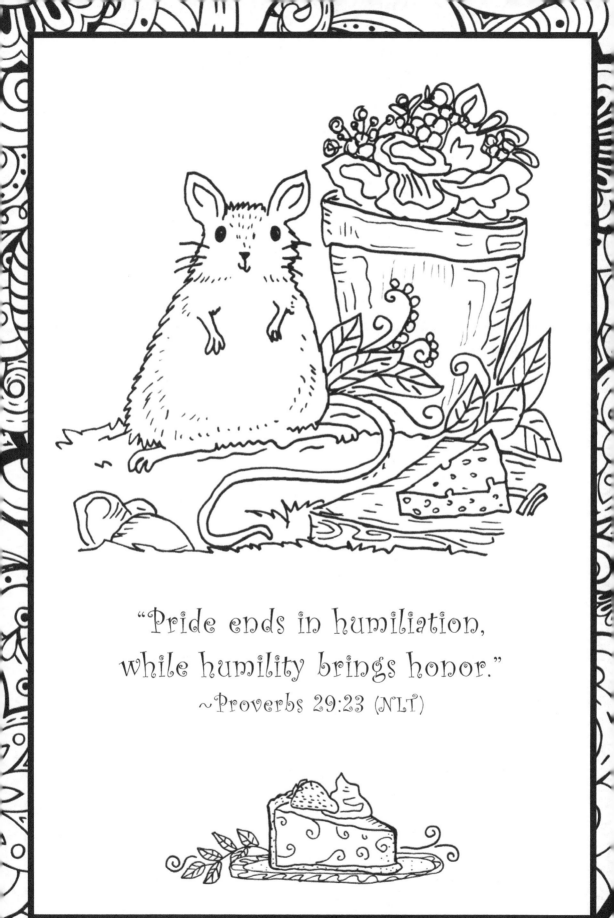

"Pride ends in humiliation,
while humility brings honor."
~Proverbs 29:23 (NLT)

Day 30 ~ Proverbs 30

"Every word of God is flawless;
*   he is a shield to those who take refuge in him.*
Do not add to his words,
*   or he will rebuke you and prove you a liar."*
                                                                ~Proverbs **30:5-6**

The first six verses of Proverbs **30** establish God as creator. The following verses, through the end of the chapter are apothegms on various subjects; two things, three things, four things. As we read the first six verses, I believe the writer is reminding us that true wisdom comes from the Lord alone. Pray before you read the Word. James **1:5** says, *"If any of you lacks wisdom, let him ask of God, who gives to all liberally and without reproach, and it will be given to him."* Pray for His understanding as you read.

"There are three things that are too amazing for me,
*   four that I do not understand:*
the way of an eagle in the sky,
*   the way of a snake on a rock,*
the way of a ship on the high seas,
*   and the way of a man with a maiden."*
                                                                ~Proverbs **30:18-19** (NIV)

If he says God's words are flawless, why does he follow with several apothegms that are too amazing to understand? I believe the writer is showing the Lord to be supreme. Pride allows man to believe we are a learned species. We have established learning institutions which hand out degrees of knowledge. Yet, even the most intelligent person who ever lived pales in comparison to the infinite knowledge of God. What is amazing is how He gives us His Word in paraphrases that are understandable on any level which can be applied to our lives thousands of years after the words were penned!

Of all the bird species, the eagle was chosen for this Proverb. If you watch an eagle soar, notice how it glides seamlessly through the air. One cannot help but marvel at its creation. We have eagles that nest close to our home. Photographers show up from all over the country to capture the elegance of their wings. Just as the writer of the Proverb, I too am amazed watching the sight of God's creation gliding through the sky. This is God's blessing to us, His encouragement.

"Who satisfies your mouth with good things,
So that your youth is renewed like the eagle's." ~Psalm **103:5**

Take time to notice the little things today. Watch a caterpillar crawl across the sidewalk. Notice the squirrels scampering about the trees. Sit for a minute and watch the fish float around the tank. Learn to take time to ponder on God's Word. Let it sink into your soul. No, in our humanness, we may not understand the "whys" of God's creation, but we can understand the deep love He has for us.
We can feel His sweet Spirit envelope our
soul.

"He encircled him, He instructed him,
He kept him as the apple of His eye.
As an eagle stirs up its nest,
Hovers over its young,
Spreading out its wings, taking them up,
Carrying them on its wings."
                    ~Deuteronomy **32:10–11**

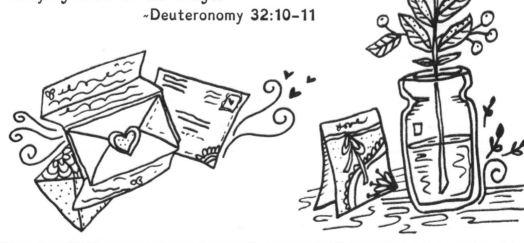

CREATIVE JOURNALING

Today's Date: _____

In Proverbs 30, which verse pops out to you? How does that verse apply to your world today? Do you take refuge in the Lord? List all the amazing little things about God:

_____
_____
_____
_____
_____
_____
_____
_____
_____
_____
_____
_____
_____
_____
_____
_____
_____
_____
_____
_____
_____
_____
_____
_____
_____
_____
_____
_____
_____

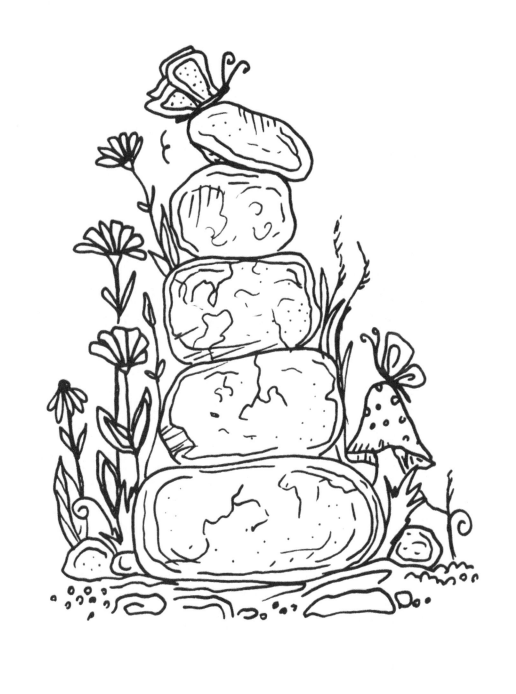

"The ants are a people not strong, yet
they prepare their food in the summer."
~Proverbs 30:25

Day 31 ~ Proverbs 31

"The words of King Lemuel,
the utterance which his mother taught him:" ~Proverbs **31:1**

When most people refer to Proverbs **31**, the *Noble Wife* is the usual commentary, describing what is commonly known as *The Virtuous Woman*. This section of the Proverbs is an interesting study as verses **10-31** are an alphabetic acrostic in Hebrew, comparable to Psalm **119**.

The first **9** verses, however, are an isolated oracle written by a mother to her son, with the counsel given by a father listed in chapter **4**. History shows the name *Lemuel* (meaning *Devoted to God*) to possibly be a name of endearment given to King Solomon by his mother, Bathsheba. Only in more modern times has the identity of the subject been questioned. Unfortunately, seeing as specific names were not given, their true origins may have been lost unto historical nonexistence.

The oracle was written as a prophetic admonition, possibly out of a mother's desire for her son's success. Most mothers' counsel is derived from past experience and a desire for their children to avoid the same mistakes made from their own life. Ironically, the three pieces of advice this mother gave were the very actions that eventually brought King Solomon to his ruin: flippant relationships, self-indulgence, and a slothful attitude toward injustice. Bathsheba would have been well equipped to warn of the consequences of these sins; the very sins of which she and King David, Solomon's father, were mercifully forgiven and restored. Centuries later, our leaders continue to embellish the same sins. We are still human. Her advice to her son, the King, could most certainly be applied not only to our government leaders of today, but to anyone in a leadership position, especially the family father.

The influential role of the mother has been greatly diminished in modern times. While the role of the father has become known for absenteeism, most people do not realize the correlation to the diminishing role of the mother. With more than a third of American households being raised by a single parent, mostly by the mother, great concern is growing over the moral decline in our society. Our children are raised without the stability of the security in a family unit, resulting in higher poverty, crime, drug usage, and lack of education. The issue is not whether the home is run by a single dad or a single mom, the issue is that neither parent is a constant in the home. Unfortunately, in modern society, most two-parent homes have two-parent incomes. The children are left to raise themselves through babysitters and day-care.

I find the addition of a woman's instruction in a man's world to be very comforting. Solomon was attributed the wisest man of all time therefore his mother's penned words must have been very influential to be included in the ancient scrolls. Never underestimate the *hand that rocks the cradle*. Most of scripture was written by men and toward men. Yet this passage contains the words of a woman giving instruction to her son, a man, a King. With such high importance placed on one oracle, it is disheartening that her words fall on deaf ears to most of our leaders today. Corruption in high places has been at work since the beginning of mankind.

"What, my son?
  And what, son of my womb?
    And what, son of my vows?" ~Proverbs **31:2**

In older translations, the chapter begins with his mother asking the question, "What?" What are you doing? Are you paying attention? Listen! Since the timeframe is not given as to when in Solomon's life the oracle was written, it is possible his mother saw in his youth warning signs of potential problems. We all have tendencies toward certain temptations. Some temptations are more common in higher positions or stations in society. This mother wished to get her son's attention to bring a warning for pitfalls of someone of his status. This mother very wisely was teaching him that the responsibility of a King is not to be taken lightly. In James **3**, we are told that teachers will receive a stricter judgment. How much more for a King? In 2nd Peter **2**, a description is given of the consequences of false teachers who lead people to destruction. Her desire was for her son to lead responsibly.

"Do not give your strength to women,
Nor your ways to that which destroys kings." ~Proverbs **31:3**

The passage gives three separate pieces of advice for successful leadership; relationship, sobriety, and advocate. The first piece of advice has been ignored by politicians and pastors alike all throughout history. Many a mighty man has fallen from the public eye due to sexual indiscretions. With the introduction of the Internet, pornography is the number one 'secret' sin of today's clergy. The temptation can be overwhelming. Bathsheba knew this first hand. Bathsheba and King David's indiscretion resulted in two deaths, a divided family, and a lost kingdom. While their hearts were forgiven and restored in relationship with God, the consequences can be felt to this day. We need to be very careful and selective with whom we are in relationship.

"It is not for kings, O Lemuel,
    It is not for kings to drink wine,
Nor for princes intoxicating drink;
    Lest they drink and forget the law,
And pervert the justice of all the afflicted.
    Give strong drink to him who is perishing,
And wine to those who are bitter of heart.
    Let him drink and forget his poverty,
And remember his misery no more." ~Proverbs **31:4-7**

The second admonition is in mind altering substances. This piece of advice should be simple common sense. But even in our society today, drunken parties for politicians are the norm. Will a people put trust in a leader who is not clear minded while they are issuing judgments, decrees, and laws? Without morality we have only chaos. Alcoholism and self-medicating are rampant. She points out that those who are perishing or are in anguish drink to forget their troubles, though her urging to give strong drink is not for a King. Her son has a greater responsibility than to be self-focused. A good King, Ruler, or

Teacher, a good Parent, is focused on those whom the Lord has put under their care. From the President/King all the way down to the parent in the poorest family, the quality of leadership is destroyed when alcohol or drugs control the mind. Just as a King is responsible for the condition of the Kingdom, Dad and Mom are responsible for the condition of the family.

"Open your mouth for the speechless,
In the cause of all who are appointed to die.
Open your mouth, judge righteously,
And plead the cause of the poor and needy." ~Proverbs **31:8-9**

The final plea this wise mother instructs her son is simply to do *good*. I believe she knew from experience within her own family how imperative righteous ruling is. James **4:17** says, *"Therefore, to him who knows to do good and does not do it, to him it is sin."* Do we sit by idly, being more concerned about our own skin, watching those under us get trampled? Do we use our position to aid those less fortunate? Most Kings and leaders throughout history succumbed to the influence of power followed by arrogance. Self-serving leaders support only those who are able to give back to their establishment or campaign. But to the little people, the poor and needy, or the unjustly charged, these leaders are mute and turn a deaf ear. Jesus said the first will be last and the last will be first. If we are in a place of position, God honors the humble in heart and giving in spirit.

Whether we are the ruler of a nation, or a stay-at-home mom, leadership comes with great responsibility. Lemuel's mother very wisely conveyed the three most important aspects of righteous leadership: stay away from physical indulgence, keep a clear head, and use the position to benefit others.

"Learn to do good;
Seek justice,
Rebuke the oppressor;
Defend the fatherless,
Plead for the widow." ~Isaiah **1:17**

CREATIVE JOURNALING

Today's Date: _____

In Proverbs **31,** which verse pops out to you? How does that verse apply to your world today? What advice would you want to convey to the next generation?

_____
_____
_____
_____
_____
_____
_____
_____
_____
_____
_____
_____
_____
_____
_____
_____
_____
_____
_____
_____
_____
_____
_____
_____
_____
_____

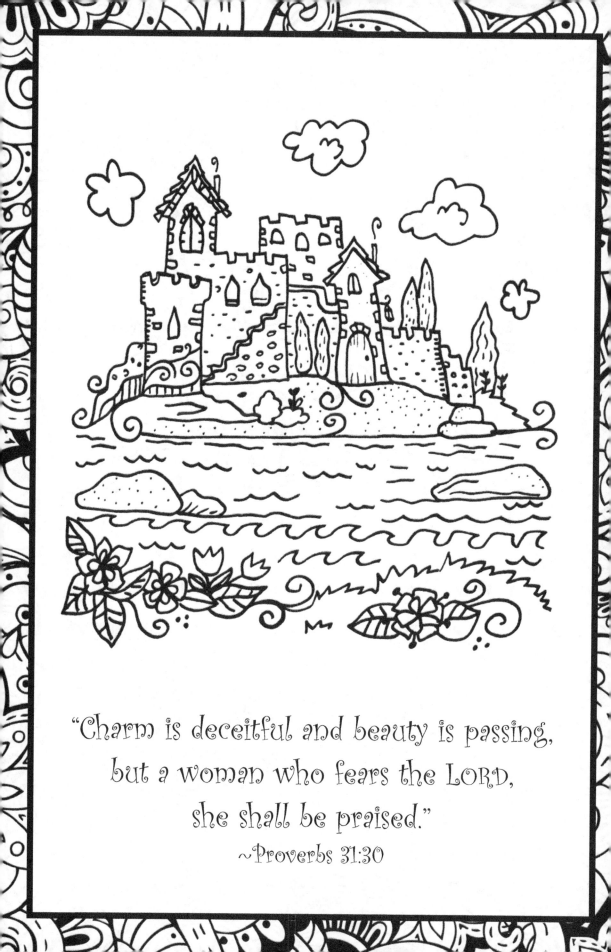

"Charm is deceitful and beauty is passing,
but a woman who fears the LORD,
she shall be praised."
~Proverbs 31:30

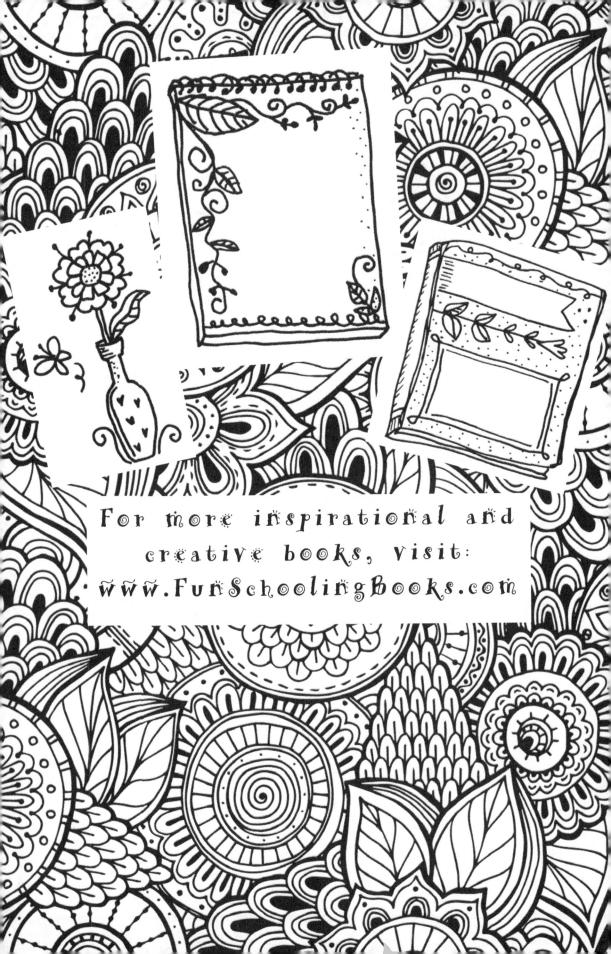

For more inspirational and creative books, visit: www.FunSchoolingBooks.com

Made in the USA
Monee, IL
10 February 2023

27458230R00077